SAVE
YOUR
KNEES

SAVE YOUR KNEES

James Fox, M.D., and Rick McGuire

A DELL TRADE PAPERBACK

Published by
Dell Publishing
a division of
Bantam Doubleday Dell Publishing Group, Inc.
666 Fifth Avenue
New York, New York 10103

Illustration on page 7 by Dr. Joel Schechter.
Illustrations on pages 10 and 30 by Dr. Joel Schechter
and Mary Ellen Thomas.
All other illustrations by Mary Ellen Thomas.

NOTE: The information contained in this book is not intended to be prescriptive. Any attempt to diagnose, treat, or rehabilitate an injury or disorder should come under the direction of a physician or orthopedic specialist.

ISBN: 0-440-50011-7

Printed in the United States of America

May 1988

10 9 8 7 6 5 4 3 2

MV

This book is dedicated to all the patients whose inglorious moments of sports and life are written across their knees and to all the people who through this book may have many more glorious moments ahead of them.

Acknowledgments

Our book and your knees owe a debt of gratitude to the efforts of a number of people. Pamela Westlin, Elizabeth Hurst, R.N., Helen Kreis, William Arnold, M.D., and Tom McGuire reviewed our manuscript and offered important comments and advice. Special thanks are also extended to those who have served as leaders, advisers, role models, and friends to the M.D.–half of this book: James Nicholas, M.D., Jack Hughston, M.D., Robert Kerlan, M.D., Frank Jobe, M.D., Jerry Kaplan, CPA, and my close friend, Mr. Danny Moscot. For the noninitialed partner, the list includes: Mrs. Patricia McGuire Atkinson, Mrs. Louise King, Mr. Clarence "Chad" Meyer, Mr. Tom Tomlinson, and the Reverend James Bortell.

One of us thanks the patients and physicians of the Southern California Orthopedic Sports Medicine Group and the other the Independent Writers of Southern California—we'll let you figure out which one thanks which.

We both owe a deep debt of gratitude to two very special contributors to this book. One is Richard "Skip" Jacobson, who spent over a hundred hours listening to this book come to life and then patiently making every word available to its readers. And the other is our editor, Jody Rein, whose suggestions contributed greatly to the usefulness of the book you hold in your hands—and the premature aging of its authors.

Finally, as the M.D. half I get the last word (my partner is much too polite since, after all, it is his keyboard): Thanks to my children, David and Lisa Fox. Having those initials after my name meant I wasn't always there physically, but I certainly was (and always will be) mentally and emotionally. Also thanks to Ellen and Karen, who each have a special place in my heart. Finally, a lifetime of thanksgiving couldn't communicate my gratitude to my mother, Helen Fox, and my late father, Max Fox, M.D., whose words of advice have lost none of their significance: "Reach beyond your grasp."

Contents

INTRODUCTION xiii

**PART ONE   WHAT'S WRONG? SYMPTOMS AND
                POSSIBLE CAUSES 1**

1

Life Is a Pain in the Knee **3**

2

On Your Knees **6**

3

There Is No Gender Gap **12**

4

Ouch! That Hurts: *From Symptoms to Diagnosis* **16**

5

What's Up, Doc? Chronic Knee Problems **26**

6

What's Up, Doc? (Revisited) Acute Knee Problems **41**

7

Arthritis: *Is It or Isn't It?* **54**

**PART TWO   WHAT TO DO ABOUT IT:
                RELIEF AND REHABILITATION 61**

8

Questions to Ask Your Doctor **63**

9

What Are You Doing to Me? **70**

10

Pain Pills and Potions **79**

11

Surgery? *The Pros and Cons* **87**

12

Arthroscopy: *Cut and Run* **90**

13

When All Else Fails: *Total Knee Replacement* **96**

14

Rehabilitation: *The Achilles' Heel of the Knee* **100**

15

Support Your Knee (*or It Won't Support You*) **118**

16

Arthritis Relief **125**

**PART THREE   BACK ON TRACK:
            SAFELY REENTERING THE
            ACTIVE WORLD   137**

17

Shoes and Orthotics: *Getting to the Foot of the Matter* **139**

18

Conditioning: *The Road to Recovery and Prevention* **147**

19

Running Scared? **155**

20

Aerobics: *The Dance of the Injured Knee* **168**

21

Skiing: *The Glide Guide* **176**

22

Basketball **189**

23

Tackling the Problems of Football **195**

24

A Six-Pack of Sports **201**

25

The Aging Athlete: *Battles of the Weekend Warrior* **222**

PART FOUR   KIDS' KNEES   227

26

What's Up, Doc? (Junior Version) **229**

27

Why Are Junior Athletics So Hazardous? **240**

EPILOGUE   KNEE NEWS IS GOOD NEWS   251

APPENDIX A   STRETCHES AND EXERCISES   259

**APPENDIX B   GLOSSARY OF ORTHOPEDIC AND
                       SPORTS MEDICINE TERMS   275**

IT CERTAINLY DOESN'T END HERE   281

INDEX   282

Introduction

"You doctors certainly have screwed up."

Me and my big mouth.

It was the spring of 1984; I was riding up a chair lift to begin a day of skiing. My whole reason for being in Utah was to relax and get away from it all; suddenly "it all" seemed to be sitting right next to me. Of course it was my own fault. I'm still a Midwestern boy at heart and I introduced myself to my seatmate. When she asked what I did for a living—I told her.

"You've really failed your patients."

"I beg your pardon."

"Just look around! It looks like a fashion show of this season's knee braces. Some are wearing those things with the big metal hinges, others have braces I've never seen before, and there are even a few Ace wraps on top of ski pants."

She paused for a breath and I noted we were too high up to jump.

"You doctors and all your fancy surgeries and high technology; the one thing you *haven't* done to your patients is educate them. You don't tell us about the risks of certain sports, you don't tell us how to strengthen our muscles so we can diminish those risks, you don't tell us the right ways to exercise, and you don't give us a clue how to prepare for major activities. Then when—surprise!—we get injured, you don't explain what happened in terms that anyone without a doctorate in physiology could understand, you don't let us in on just what all that fancy equipment of yours is supposed to be doing to us, and you end up just sending us back out to get hurt again.

"Doctors should be more than technicians," she said with a hint of finality that unfortunately wasn't to materialize for several thousand feet yet. "You should be teachers."

The lecture continued for the remaining seven minutes up the mountain, then she took off down the slopes. I stood atop the run, looked out over a breathtaking expanse of mountain wilderness, and my first thought was "What a way to start a beautiful day of skiing." My second thought was "You know, she's right."

In defense, may I note that this wasn't the first time that I recognized the problem. When I was a resident in orthopedic training in New York City, it became obvious to me that there were marked limitations to our medical program, especially as it related to knees. I'd had a number of patients come to me with injured knees, including such things as torn ligaments, arthritic problems, and tears of the menisci. In reviewing the available literature, there were fascinating reports of whole new approaches to knee problems, and we appeared to be on the edge of some major medical advancements, but little of this had crossed over yet into day-to-day practice. Because I felt so strongly that this was the future of orthopedics, I made a concerted effort to get involved. I was fortunate, through the American Academy of Orthopedic Surgeons Sports Medicine Committee, to be selected for the first Fellowship in Sports Medicine in Orthopedics.

My enthusiasm for the knee remains. It's perhaps the most vulnerable piece of the anatomy; it certainly wasn't designed with modern sports and activities in mind! However, we are finally starting to get a real feel for how the knee properly operates—and what to do when it doesn't.

Within the last ten years our understanding of the knee and our ability to treat it has increased so fast that researchers can't disseminate the news fast enough to the medical profession, let alone to the public. This has left us with an education gap the size of the Grand Canyon.

So, today, my private practice is dedicated solely to the knee. My

weekends over much of the year are spent participating in confer-
ences where I lecture and teach before orthopedic surgeons and
practitioners. My partners and I founded the Center for Disorders of
the Knee and each year the institute publishes several dozen articles
or research papers. We also recognized the need for patient education several years ago, and that's when we designed a series of
video tapes, brochures, and even a newsletter to help our patients
recover from their sports medicine problems.

However, my chair-lift partner's criticisms were justified. When I
returned to the Los Angeles area, I went to a number of bookstores
searching racks and shelves for sports medicine literature, and what
I learned is that according to the popular press, today's athletic
body consists of a back and something that's apparently feeding it.
You can take your sports medicine in the form of sports nutrition
and bad backs; beyond that, we're apparently in great shape. Then
why is it that the knee is the number one problem facing orthopedic
surgeons?

Anyone who reads the sports pages, watches athletics on television, or hears the sports report on radio is aware of the high
frequency of knee injuries. What hasn't been recognized, at least
not by the mass media, is that knee problems certainly aren't
confined to professional athletes. According to a Harris Poll, one
out of two American adults exercises regularly, and medical experts
say one out of ten of them suffers a sports-related injury each year.
The annual cost of these injuries, including hospital bills, physical
therapy sessions, and hours lost from work exceeds $40 billion!
And study after study shows that in most activities, the number-one
site of injury is the knee.

When my fruitless search of the popular literature was over, I
began to ask various people what they needed to know to understand their knees better, not just to understand what their doctor
was telling them but also to really understand what happened to
them and how they could avoid having it happen to them again.
From these conversations it became obvious that people need to
understand how the knee is constructed, the function of ligaments,
bones, and cartilage, the particular problems which even the best
knees are heir to, and the best solutions that are presently available.
There is also a deep concern about communication: How do I

understand what my doctor is saying? How do I get him or her to understand what *I* am saying? And (to get to real basics) how do I find a doctor?

With the problem delineated and the task before me, I teamed up with Rick McGuire, one of the leading health and medical writers in the country. Together we've tried to answer the basic questions asked by anyone with a knee problem. We take a look at the problems and symptoms associated with knees; we guide you through the recovery process and then we look at a wide variety of sports and activities to help you avoid a painful reprise.

Although this book is written to give you a highly readable cover-to-cover account of knees and knee problems, the chapters are designed to give you quick access to whatever information you're looking for. Do you want to know about symptoms, treatment, surgery, or exercises? Turn to that part of the chapter. If you want to see what you need to do to get your knees back in fit form, turn to the appendix, prop the book open, and find a space to work your legs. And if you want to know what to ask your doctor when you limp into the examination room, there's a list of questions you can take with you.

All in all, you're about to learn the inside story about life in a real joint; fortunately, it's not as frightening as it seems. I promise it won't hurt. In fact, I think you'll be relieved when you learn just what's going on in there. Prop your legs up on a comfortable stool and get started.

And if you're ever next to me on a chair lift as we start out for a day of skiing, don't tell *me* I haven't done anything to save your knees!

PART ONE

What's Wrong?
Symptoms and Possible Causes

1

Life Is a Pain in the Knee

Of the 187 joints in the body, the knee is, without a doubt, the best at grabbing one's attention. Everyone who has ever misjudged a doorway, opened a door while standing in its path, or kneed a piece of furniture has the feel of an angry knee clearly in mind.

That's because the knee is the most vulnerable joint in the body and that's why bum knees are endemic to active America. Nearly half a million knee surgeries are performed each year in the United States. Knee symptoms are the number one reason people visit orthopedic surgeons. Complain about an aching knee and you'll find plenty of company. An estimated 50 million Americans have suffered or are suffering knee pain or injuries. And if you want to feel better about your own knee, just bring up the subject in front of two or more people. Odds are that one of them will have a knee story that will make your knees buckle.

For an estimated 17 million athletes, the injury rate in such sports as football, gymnastics, skiing, and racket sports is projected at over 50 percent. Guess what's injured the most? According to sports medicine specialists, the initial complaint of over half the athletes they see is knee pain. If you're an athlete, the chances of knee surgery are five times greater than surgery on any other part of your body. Just ask Joe Namath, Bobby Orr, Gale Sayers, or Mickey Mantle about knee problems. More recently the Injured Knee Hall of Pain has welcomed Phil Esposito, Dan Marino, Bernard King, and Gary Carter. For all their touchdowns, goals, and home runs, these players will also be remembered for their shattered knees.

Thousands of others have their own personal memories of fiery pain and smoldering injuries: Between 1961 and 1970, 70 percent of all football players had knee surgery by the age of twenty-six, including half of all running backs and virtually every quarterback. In 1984, 38 percent of all players on the NFL's injured reserve list were there because of knee injuries. And when the National Collegiate Athletic Association surveyed seven sports, they found that the knee was the most common injury site.

The part-time athlete is also susceptible to a host of orthopedic injuries. According to a Harris Poll, one of every two American adults exercise regularly, and medical experts say one out of ten of them suffers a sports-related injury each year. In San Francisco a sports medicine clinic recently reviewed 10,000 recreational injuries, and nine activities—basketball, dance, football, gymnastics, running, skiing, tennis, soccer, and figure skating—accounted for three fourths of the injuries. What part of the anatomy was number one on the hit parade? Knees. In fact, looking at the incidence of injury to each part of the body, for most sports, injuries to the knee were more common than the next three injury sites combined.

This epidemic of strains, sprains, and tears is, at least in part, a by-product of the widespread interest in aerobic conditioning. It's hard to argue against something that is such a major advance in general health and fitness, but a physiologist recently noted, "A strong cardiovascular system doesn't do you much good when the other parts of your body are shot to hell."

Of course you certainly don't have to be athletic to learn more than you ever wanted to know about knee pain. What's the most dangerous place for a knee outside of sports? Inside an automobile, attached to someone who hasn't fastened his or her seat belt. Nearly one out of every three car-accident injuries is to the knee. Even if you always buckle up, a car can be no friend of knees; you can open a door on one, or even twist it just getting in or out.

Other places hazardous to the health of a knee include work, the home, and the world in general. Whether you're climbing a flight of stairs, scrubbing a floor, trying to navigate a slippery sidewalk, or just out dancing, there are accidents waiting to happen to your knees.

Why are we so knee deep in injury? Well, quite frankly, when God designed the knee, He (or She) certainly wasn't thinking of modern living. The knee is the largest, most unstable, and perhaps most complicated joint in the human body. For many of the demands we place on our knees, we need a joint that's rugged, like the hip, which is a ball and socket design with inherent stability. Instead, we get two giant bones propped on top of one another, held together by the anatomical equivalent of rubber bands. Yet this delicate apparatus is expected to function flawlessly through all manner of self-inflicted trauma—jogging, jumping, skiing, skating, training, and straining. That's a lot to ask of a joint designed two and a half million years ago for an animal that wasn't even walking upright at the time!

While it's true that injuries to the knee have received more attention in the medical literature over the past ten years than injuries to any other joint in the body, there is a downside to all this information. The art of treating the knee has advanced so rapidly that orthopedists are hard pressed to keep up with the variety of injuries and instabilities they are learning to diagnose and define. Fortunately, some of the greatest advances have come in the area of prevention. Unfortunately, few people make an appointment with their doctor at least one week prior to injury in order to discuss prevention.

This shortsighted approach to knee care and maintenance is one reason behind the development of this book. Consider this a preventive-medicine house call. Whether you're a novice at knee pain or an old pro at hobbling around, this is what you need to know to save your knees.

However, in order to fully understand and utilize the knee-saving benefits of this book, a little anatomy is necessary. Although high school biology may have made you cringe, the easy background presented next is guaranteed to be a lot less painful than the trauma you may face without this information!

2

On Your Knees

Once the knee was considered little more than a basic hinge; like a garden gate, it swung open and closed. This reductionist view was eagerly embraced by the medical profession, which had enough problems to contend with without worrying about a joint that seemed to be simplicity in motion. However, it offered little comfort to patients who were in agonizing pain.

Today we recognize that the knee doesn't just flex; it also glides, slides, twists, rocks, and rolls. The demands placed upon the modern knee would be a challenge to the best-designed machine, but the knee is the most poorly constructed joint in the body, with little intrinsic stability. Consequently, almost everything people do for recreation is tough on the knee. In fact, much of what the knee faces in simple day-to-day living—kneeling, walking, climbing, and being crossed while at rest—can take a toll over time.

At its most fundamental, the knee is indeed a hinge that connects the thighbone (*femur*) and the leg bone (*tibia*). While seated, the bones barely touch, but stand up and they lock together, providing a strong, unified structure.

Holding these two bones together are four major ligaments: the two *collateral* ligaments, which run up the inside and outside of the leg, and the two *cruciate* (as in "excruciating pain") ligaments, which cross within the joint. The former provide side-to-side stabil-

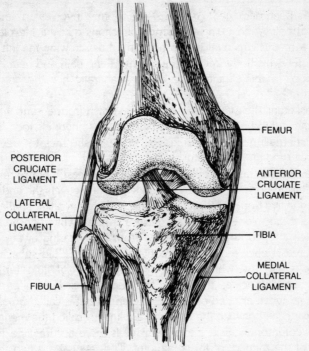

The collateral and cruciate ligaments

ity, while the latter prevent the bones from slipping backward or forward out of the joint. No matter how powerful the muscles around the knee, without most of its strong, resilient ligaments, the joint would be useless.

The *anterior* (front-to-back) *cruciate ligament* (ACL) is often torn in contact sports or sprained during activity. Like its partner, the *posterior* (back-to-front) *cruciate ligament* (PCL), it should look like a good strong rope. However, when it's torn completely, it becomes a frayed mass swaying in the currents. Some athletes can get by without it, others need a knee brace or surgery.

The primary problem with ligaments is that they are tough but not particularly flexible. Once stretched, a ligament tends to stay stretched, and if stretched beyond 6 percent of its length, it snaps, leaving the knee vulnerable to further injury.

If an audible "pop" is noted upon injury, the odds are that the

ACL has been damaged. A classic ACL rupture involves an athlete who is running and trying to change directions quickly. He plants his left foot and cuts over it with his right, thus screwing the left leg as he rotates his body until he feels excruciating pain and hears the knee pop. In this situation the athlete generally hits the ground before the ball does.

In basketball the player may be coming down from a jump when he or she is thrown off balance by landing on someone's foot. The femur externally rotates and extends as he or she tries to prevent falling, causing an ACL rupture.

Bones are soft enough to wear away with the least bit of rubbing, so to alleviate bone-on-bone wear and tear nature covers the ends of the most active bones with a natural shock absorber called *cartilage*. There are no blood vessels or nerves in this white, gristle-like substance and, to keep this cartilage from just wearing away, the whole area is enclosed in a sac containing a thick fluid substance that looks like the white of an egg. This *synovial* fluid further protects and lubricates the joint. The sac itself is known as the *bursa*, and when irritated over time, the end result is called *bursitis*.

The cartilage between the bones in the knee is called the *menisci*. What is commonly called a torn cartilage is more accurately a tear of one of the menisci of the knee joint. The menisci are two thin, crescent-shaped structures that act as shock absorbers between the thigh and leg bones. By pushing synovial fluid around, they also contribute to the lubrication of the knee and to the nourishment of the cartilage. A child's ability to jump for joy, a professional athlete's career, and an elderly person's general mobility all largely depend on the way the cartilage crumbles.

There are two basic types of meniscal tears: acute tears and degenerative tears. (For detailed information, see Chapter 6.) Originally, orthopedic surgeons felt that any torn meniscus must be totally removed. Indeed, during the sixties and seventies meniscectomy was the most common orthopedic surgical procedure. Now we realize that he who hesitates is saved. Looking back on all those meniscectomies, we discovered that people who have a torn meniscus removed in their twenties have a greatly increased risk of developing *arthritis* by the time they're forty-five or fifty. In fact, studies have found evidence of degenerative changes within the knee in up to 85 percent of meniscectomy patients at a ten-year follow-up. What this means for all those athletes who had meniscectomies during the 1950s, 1960s, and early 1970s remains to be seen. Unfortunately, the feeling in the sports medicine community is that, due to those meniscectomies, the number of former athletes who will need total knee replacement will increase steadily during the next couple of decades.

This is because without the meniscus acting as a buffer, the two joint bones rub against each other. In time the bones can wear away at the ends, leaving nerves painfully exposed. The result is *osteoarthritis,* or degenerative arthritis, which can spread to the entire joint.

Researchers estimate that the medial meniscus and anterior cruciate ligament absorb 90 percent of all knee injuries. Once they were a primary cause of lifelong limps. Today if the injured is lucky and the injury is accurately diagnosed, he or she will be left with little more than a dot of a scar and an heroic tale of medical trauma to entertain the masses or at least the folks at the next cocktail party.

The mode of injury for the meniscus is similar to that of the ACL. Often they are injured together and that can confuse all concerned. If one problem and not the other is corrected, the knee is still damaged and very susceptible to reinjury.

Moving on, the front shield of the knee is the ever-popular kneecap or *patella.* When you knee a piece of furniture or open a door without getting out of the way, it is the kneecap that lets you know you've made a mistake. The patella moves within a track near the end of the thighbone. A severe sudden twist or constant stress can throw the kneecap off track. Although it takes some powerful abuse, when it is seriously injured it can take much of the future with it.

That's because the kneecap is the fulcrum that gives power to the muscles of the leg. It also absorbs a lot of the stress of daily activities, like climbing stairs. You don't realize it, but when you simply walk up a few stairs the pressures across your knees are approximately four times your body weight! This massive load is largely due to forces that are generated by muscles being worked. Furthermore, damage to any major muscle in the leg will mean more work for the patella and could begin to wear it down.

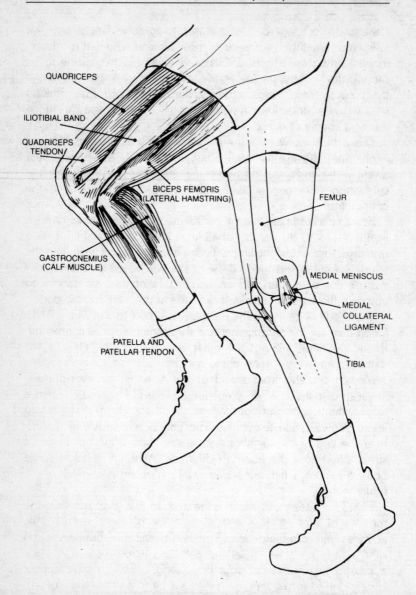

The major muscles and bones of the knee and legs

Tying all this together is a thick and powerful system of muscles and tendons that flex, drive, and support the knee. The front thigh (quadriceps), hamstring, and calf muscles are the three major muscle groups involved and the only supporting structures that can be strengthened. The patella tendon connects the kneecap to the front thigh muscle and shinbone. A tear here is called "jumper's knee" and is common among basketball and volleyball players, hurdlers, and male dancers.

Injury to any of these structures, which provide stability at the knee joint, represents a major cause of disability, loss of playing time, and the beginning of the degenerative arthritic changes that may befall an active individual.

If all of this makes you feel like wearing designer armor the next time you're heading out for a little recreation, do remember that probably 70 percent of all knee injuries are of a relatively minor nature. And you'll be much better equipped to both prevent and pinpoint your own knee problems now that you know what's where!

3

There Is No Gender Gap

Training and locker rooms were once largely "Men Only," but not anymore. In fact, while women make up 52 percent of the population, they comprise 60 percent of the nation's health-club memberships.

Not surprisingly, along with this increase in activity there has been an increase in sports-related injuries suffered by women. The big question causing considerable debate within sports medicine circles has to do with the relative risks women face in sports activities: Are women at more risk of injury than men?

At the present time this is pretty swampy medical ground and home to some pretty muddy statistics. But what are the sporting facts of life? Well, women do tend to sustain more injuries than men. For example, after reviewing the injuries sustained by male and female basketball teams during two consecutive seasons, researchers from Northwestern University Medical School, Chicago, found that women sustained 60 percent more injuries than the men.

In their paper, which was published in *The American Journal of Sports Medicine* (10:5, 297–99, 1982), the authors reported that both sexes had similar ankle injury rates (which was the most frequently injured body part), but the women incurred considerably more knee and thigh injuries as well as more sprains, strains, and contusions. Women are at a greater risk, apparently. Now the question is whether or not their added risk of injury is based on inherent differences between the sexes. To answer this question we first need to know what the real differences are that would affect sports performance and if these differences are really to blame for women's injuries.

We do know that women tend to be more flexible than men, which is good because this can mean fewer muscular difficulties. However, the characteristics of the female body often breed trouble. Women may be predisposed to knee injuries because their wider hips cause their major leg bone, the femur, to turn slightly inward, putting more pressure on delicate knee joints. This wider pelvis and angling thighbone may lead to a number of problems, including a chronic condition known as runner's knee, in which the kneecap shifts sideways and rubs against nearby cartilage. This extra width at the hips can also cause a stretching of the quadriceps muscles, which leads to tendon and knee pain. Finally, women in general have only 80 percent of the muscle mass that men do, so pound for pound there is less muscle support for the knee.

Are these differences reflected in actual injury rates, like those uncovered by the Northwestern University researchers? Many experts believe that they are, but like everyone else, experts can make perfect sense and still be wrong.

For years we've known that among women's sports, basketball has the highest injury rate. This isn't terribly surprising, considering that men's basketball has the highest injury rate among noncollision collegiate sports. However, studies have suggested that female players sustain more injuries, lose more time while they recover, and require surgery more frequently than male basketball players.

When this problem was first recognized, several investigators concluded that women's knees were not as tight as men's knees and this added laxity meant a greater predisposition to injury. However, we now know that there is no significant difference between the knee laxity of males and females.

Other researchers thought that the added risk might be due to women's smaller ligaments or perhaps to those biomechanical differences we mentioned. While these factors haven't been dismissed, a more likely candidate for blame has been found: inadequate conditioning.

How conditioning (or lack thereof) takes its toll is best explained by a study comparing injuries sustained by two Oklahoma City varsity basketball teams (*The Physician and Sportsmedicine*, 6:10, 92–95, 1978). While the boys' team showed a consistent rate of injury throughout the season, the members of the girls' team were about six times as likely to be injured in the first three months of the season compared to the last two months of play, when their injury rate was nearly identical to the boys' team. This suggests that the girls were in poorer condition at the start of the season, so they were injured frequently until they were conditioned and more experienced.

A study released just as this book was going into production confirms the importance of conditioning and adds another element for injury prevention. The National Athletic Trainers' Association (NATA) in June of 1987 reported the results of the first nationwide survey of injuries among girls who play high school basketball. They found that 23 percent of the more than 400,000 girls playing the game were sidelined at least once during the preceding school year. Their recommendations for curbing the injury rate: Improve physical conditioning programs and institute a five-minute warm-up period after halftime. The latter suggestion was based on the fact that fully 60 percent of all game-related injuries occurred during the second half of the play. Many of these injuries could be prevented, according to NATA, by simple stretching and flexibility exercises prior to the start of the second half.

So in reviewing the available literature (which is none too extensive), women may be inherently more susceptible than men to muscular injuries due to a difference in muscle mass. And, due to their overall alignment, women may be at greater risk of knee problems in general. On the other hand, women may not be as likely to sustain a ligamentous injury. However, most of the injury rate difference between men and women in sports could be erased with improved strengthening and conditioning programs for women.

There may be other factors influencing women's injury rates in sports, but it may be a while before these are revealed. The problem is that we're not sure yet how much of what we're learning is true and how much is statistical aberration.

If you're concerned about being injured in your chosen sporting endeavors, whether you're a pro or a rank (or unranked) amateur, you largely create your own risk of injury by choosing how prepared you are for action. Want to avoid injury? A good place to start would be to incorporate the protective stretching and conditioning exercises at the end of this book into your activity schedule.

Here's some encouraging news: in the November 1984 issue of *The Journal of Musculoskeletal Medicine,* when highly trained athletes are compared, there is no difference in injury rates between the sexes. This means that as opportunities open up and better conditioning and training programs are initiated for women, the rate of injury to women should continue to decline.

4
Ouch! That Hurts:
From Symptoms to Diagnosis

Of course the obvious question is how do you know if your injury requires medical attention or if it can be brought around with a little verbal exercise and some T.L.C.?

The key is understanding what your knee is trying to tell you. It's hard to be a conscientious care-giver if you haven't a clue as to what your charge is saying. With a better understanding of symptoms, you'll be a much better guardian to your knee and a lot better patient for your doctor.

In 1985 over 650,000 patients underwent arthroscopy for diagnosis and repair of knee injuries, 84,000 patients had ligamentous repairs, and another 75,000 people were fitted with artificial knees. If these figures make you weak in the knees, the good news is that the vast majority of knee injuries do not require surgical intervention.

From the doctor's perspective, this is good; any time you invade the body, even for a relatively benign procedure, there is the possibility of complications. Unfortunately, the high-tech advancements of the last few years have gotten a lot of attention, and as a result, particularly for the sports-minded, surgery has become the instant panacea for all known knee ills. That's not a healthy attitude. There is no orthopedic condition that cannot be made worse by surgery. Yet, to most people, the knee is an absolute mystery. Well, we've gone through some of the cast of characters. Now it's time to start reading your knee. The plot thickens.

EFFUSION, or SWELLING

The pressure of local swelling, or effusion, is one of the most common knee symptoms. This is nature's way of limiting knee activity until healing occurs or the mechanical disability that is causing the swelling is corrected surgically.

To your doctor, swelling occurs when excess fluid accumulates *outside* of a joint. If the fluid gathers *within* a joint, the problem is said to be *effusion*. If you report swelling, 98 percent of the time the problem is caused by effusion. In other words, "swelling" has both a technical meaning and a layman's meaning. However, we give up. There's no point in bucking that kind of a tide. So, in this book we'll use the term swelling and not effusion.

There are two types of swelling: One is caused by an increase in the production of the knee's own lubricant, synovial fluid, and the other by blood where it doesn't belong (hemarthrosis). If the swelling occurs within the first hour of injury, there is probably bleeding into the joint. If it takes longer, the joint is frantically pumping out additional fluid into the synovial lining trying to lubricate an abnormality within the knee.

Sudden and Intermediate Swelling

Sudden swelling within an hour or so of the injury is very suggestive of bleeding into the joint and is probably a ligamentous tear (most often of the anterior cruciate ligament) or a fracture. Swelling that occurs anywhere from two to twenty-four hours after an injury is more likely to be a tear of the meniscus, most commonly medial meniscus. If the knee blows up suddenly and then decompresses, that's no time to relax. It could mean major ligamentous damage and injuries involving multiple ligaments around the knee. Indeed, you may have just managed to blow out all the major structures in the knee, including the surrounding envelope, which allows fluid to rush out and bleed into the fatty tissue beneath the skin. That's why it swells and decompresses so fast. Normal swelling can be compared to a dam with a slow leak. But in the case of a pedestrian accident where the knee is struck by a car bumper, a major skiing accident, or any high-velocity/high-force injury, it's more like a dam that breaks and floods the countryside.

The best home treatment for swelling is RICE—rest, ice, compression with a light wrap, and elevation. The immediate application of ice (not directly on skin but wrapped in a towel) can limit the extent of tissue damage and shorten healing time considerably. However, with swelling that occurs two to six hours later, ice is not as beneficial.

Chronic Swelling

If swelling is a problem of long-standing, the individual may describe his condition as *water on the knee.* The most likely cause is a mechanical or internal derangement caused by trauma, such as a meniscal tear, a knee sprain, or a ruptured ligament. (In children's knees the causes of swelling are likely to be quite different. See Chapter 26.) Probably the single most important factor in determining the cause of swelling is a careful review of just what the knee was doing at the time in question. Swelling can sneak up on you, in which case it could be related to arthritis, loose bodies knocking around inside the knee, or infection. If the swelling is rapid, trauma, no matter how trivial, is likely to be the cause. Squatting and turning, or simply turning with the knee flexed and the foot planted, can be enough to tear a meniscus.

If ignored, swelling distends the knee, prohibits full range of motion, and muscles may atrophy from non-use. Furthermore, if the effusion is caused by internal bleeding, the blood acts as a destructive irritant. It may be hard to imagine blood inside the body as an irritant—it's hard to think of air as an irritant either until the dentist blows it on a cavity. Iron within the blood especially irritates the lining of the knee and can even become deposited on the joint surfaces.

Sometimes the only way to get rid of this excess fluid is to drain it off by needle aspiration. If the swelling is easily explained by the circumstances of the injury, a needle aspiration for diagnostic purposes may not be necessary. However, sometimes a sample of the fluid does need to be analyzed for infection, the presence of *gout, pseudo-gout,* or arthritis. If fat droplets are found suspended in the fluid, this suggests that a bone has fractured.

Sometimes anti-inflammatory agents, such as aspirin, are given to decrease the swelling, but it should be remembered that knees don't just swell for the fun of it. A swollen knee has a serious problem and it's telling you that it needs medical attention.

Problem	Degree of Swelling (3 is most)	Speed of Onset	Other Symptoms	Method of Injury
Meniscal tear	1–2	2–8 hrs.	Locked knee Pain Tearing sensation	Twisting or squatting
Sprains Grade 1 Grade 2 Grade 3	1 2–3 3	Immediate	Severe pain Instability	Falls Twisting injuries
Chondromalacia patella	1	Slow and insidious	Aching on front of knee Pseudo-locking Instability Pain with flexion	Subluxated patella Repetitive squatting Overweight Blunt trauma
Osteochondritis dissecans	1	Slow and insidious	Pseudo-locking Low-grade aching Weakness Loose bodies	Unknown
Loose body	2	Intermittent	True locking Instability	Sheer fractures Osteochondritis dissecans
Osteoarthritis	1–2	Slow and insidious	Stiffness Low-grade aching	Old trauma Aging process
Rheumatoid arthritis	2–3	Slow and insidious	Stiffness Loss of movement Low-grade aching	Unknown
Gout and pseudo-gout	2	2–6 hours	Limited movement	Metabolic disease

LOCKING

There are two types of locking, true locking and *pseudo-locking*. More precisely, there's what your doctor would call locking and what you would describe as locking.

True Locking

For the orthopedist, true locking doesn't mean that the knee can't be moved, but rather that something is preventing it from fully straightening out. It's like trying to close a door that's wedged open. Whatever it is that's wedged in there may slide out of the way (only to remind you of its presence by sliding back again when you least expect it) or it may be a source of continuing trauma.

The key to locking is often a torn cartilage or a loose body (such as a bone chip) that has finally been caught and it has grabbed your attention. The locking of a meniscus, at least on the first occasion, generally occurs while doing something active, like playing football. A loose body lock is more likely to occur during an everyday activity, such as walking downstairs.

"How come I have this torn cartilage and it locked on me and I've never had a major injury?" I hear patients complain. If pressed, some do recall some sort of injury, maybe twenty years ago, but it was "no big deal." That loose body in your knee may have been off to the side, with everything functioning fine, until that one additional maneuver gave it just enough freedom to get caught. Or perhaps there truly was no one traumatic incident that initiated the whole process. Imagine a carpenter who is constantly squatting. For whatever reason, every time this carpenter squats there is a tear of his cartilage, microscopic at first, then after two years it's a millimeter wide, another two years and another millimeter of tear, and finally one day it rips completely.

If the problem is a loose body sailing around the synovial sea, it probably started off as a small bone chip that broke loose during a moment of trauma. They range from sand size to as large as a quarter. Of course the body doesn't like UFO's (Unidentified Floating Objects), so it tries to break them down and reabsorb them. If that doesn't work, it tries to wall the intruder off by laying down scar tissue, or it may start laying calcium over it. In either case the end result is felt as a locking sensation or a "giving way" of the knee.

To alleviate true locking, the fragment must be removed, whether it's a bone chip or a torn meniscus. Otherwise there will be subsequent damage as the fragment continues to wedge itself into the bones of the knee. Fortunately, bothersome pieces of cartilage can easily be removed by a surgical technique called arthroscopy. (See Chapter 12.)

Some people have tried rest, elevation, and anti-inflammatories in an attempt to lesson the swelling that sometimes accompanies locking. Occasionally this allows the fragment to slide back into place. Others have also tried twisting or manipulating the leg. However, the best answer is still a surgical one.

Pseudo-locking

The second type, which I call pseudo-locking, is what a lot of people call locking when certain movements simply hurt too much to do. The knee may not be incapable of complete movement, but there is an area of exposed surface within the knee. When that surface bumps up against another surface there is pain and discomfort, which discourages you from extending your knee all the way.

So you tell your doctor your knee is locked and you can't straighten your leg out all the way. You say, "My knee locked while going down a flight of stairs. There was this sharp pain and then I couldn't move it." I say, "But can you move it if you try?" "Yes," you say, "but it hurts." What is actually happening is that when your knee hits a particular angle or feels a certain pressure, it hits the panic button, triggering protective muscle function and a string of internal expletives.

The most common cause is damage to the knee surface, generally *chondromalacia patella* or osteoarthritis. You will likely have a history of grating within the knee if you develop pseudo-locking. You're also a likely victim of a subluxating or dislocating patella. Swelling, however, is not common.

For pseudo-locking the best treatment is rest, which allows the area of irritation to heal and then regain its movement and strength. So if you suffer from an episode of pseudo-locking, relax. Get off your feet for a few minutes. Usually you'll be able to move again—gently—after a few minutes. A cold pack while you're resting may also help.

GIVING WAY

Sometimes a knee doesn't lock, but it does give way for a moment, giving the owner a bit of a stop. When I was growing up in the Midwest I had an electric train. If it went over an imperfect junction it would bounce off the edge and bump right back onto the track. Like my Lionel train, the knee has three tracks. One holds the kneecap (or patella). If, for some reason, the kneecap doesn't stay in its track and *subluxates* (slips out) for a moment, your thigh muscles lose control. That's instability. If one of my Lincoln logs fell across my train track, it would derail. A loose body along the general track of your knee probably won't derail you, but you'll know you've hit a bump. And the third track is made up of your ligaments. Perhaps they've been damaged by injury or become stretched out. The forces of movement may be too much for them to handle and they give way. All of these would come under the general diagnosis of patella subluxation or dislocation.

Another possibility is that the muscles that control the knee are weak and unstable; perhaps there was a previous injury and they have not been properly rehabilitated. If the muscles lose control for a moment, you feel them give way and you instinctively reach for support or prepare for a fall.

Giving way due to an old ligament injury, muscle instability, or the locking of a loose body frequently occurs while descending stairs or jumping from a height. If the problem is a torn cartilage, the triggering event is often a rotary movement, such as turning round suddenly, stepping on a small stone, or walking on uneven ground.

SNAP, CRACKLE, POP

Perhaps the most common concern expressed about the knee comes from people who worry about the snap, crackle, and pop that comes with activity. They fear that their knees are deteriorating right before their very ears. For the most part, as long as there is no accompanying pain, an occasional grumble from the knee should not be of major concern. In fact, considering what the joint is forced to put up with over the course of daily living, it's not all that surprising that most people over the age of twenty manage to hear at least some knee noise.

Generally, such sounds can be traced to tiny bits of cartilage that have chipped away from bone and gone floating off into the synovial sea. When the joint moves, the chip passes between the intact cartilage and makes a popping sound. Usually, this is not painful and does not damage the joint. It just makes it tricky to sneak up on people.

When large pieces of cartilage have broken off, however, they may actually chip away more protective cartilage as they go popping around the knee. And if a large piece wedges itself between the bones, the knee may suddenly lock.

How can you tell if the sounds you hear are just normal Rice Krispies or something more serious? Sometimes it's difficult. If you're concerned about it, see your orthopedic specialist. However, the rule of thumb (or knee) is that you're safe as long as there is no accompanying pain, swelling, or loss of function. For example, if you can't sit for a normal length of time without pain, that would indicate a loss of function. (That's what the British call "the theater sign.") If you have poorly localized knee pain, which is exacerbated by going down stairs and hills, that also could indicate a more serious problem. Again, when in doubt, ask a specialist.

Most commonly heard is an occasional click, which is fairly universal and represents nothing very significant. Too many clicks, however, equal a creak, and you don't want to be up a creek without a diagnosis. So if you're worried, check in for a checkup.

The most common cause of all this noise is chondromalacia patella, which results from trauma. A subluxating or dislocating patella is also a possibility, with traumatic and degenerative arthritis a less likely competitor in the snap, crackle, pop diagnostic derby.

A snap or pop (which is not accompanied by a traumatic event) could represent something sliding over the joint, such as a torn cartilage or a loose fragment. It could also be the kneecap snapping or popping along (or out of) its track.

Crackling, grating, or grinding is most worrisome. That is called crepitation, and it means that there is a roughness to a surface and you're hearing bone rubbing against bone or roughened cartilage. That's a much more ominous sign of degeneration of a joint surface.

PAIN AND TENDERNESS

Pain may be caused by swelling, nerve fibers that have become torn or irritated, or degenerative changes, most often associated with arthritis. If you can accurately locate the site of the pain, it will greatly assist the doctor in making the diagnosis. Of course if you happen to be a procrastinator, it's best to remember where the pain was felt first.

The location of the pain, the severity of the pain, and what makes the pain occur all offer clues to the underlying problem. For example, a low-grade aching pain on the front of the knee occurring during hill climbing most likely represents chondromalacia patella. The same pain may also appear in the middle of physical activity and the same patella problem is probably at fault. (For more information concerning this and other specific complaints, please hobble over to Chapter 5.)

Such low-grade pain often begins after activity, but if you persist in these activities, the pain becomes sharper and more persistent. If left untreated, the pain may eventually force you to severely restrict your activity. Besides chondromalacia patella, this type of pain is symptomatic with *tendinitis, patellar tendinitis,* or stress fractures on the front of the knee and *iliotibial band friction syndrome* on the outer side of the knee or bursitis on the inner side.

Another classic pain is often quite sharp and associated with a tearing sensation, swelling, and instability, all brought about thanks to a fall or twisting maneuver deep within the knee. Such moves can cause either ligament or meniscal damage. The mode of injury is often an athlete attempting to change direction quickly. If there is an audible "Pop!" upon injury, the problem is likely to be a torn anterior cruciate ligament. If the pain occurs on either side of the knee, then the injury is suggestive of a medial (inner) or lateral (outer) ligament or meniscus tear.

PUTTING IT ALL TOGETHER

Let's take an example and look at what happens to a knee, and to add some drama to the script, let's say your first response is to ignore the problem. (Sound at all familiar?) Your foot is planted and you make a sudden turn. No big deal, a little swelling perhaps. But a part of your meniscus has torn and it's caught there between the inner edge of your femur and tibia. You continue to walk on it, trying to force the knee closed with every step. Your knee says, "This is stupid. If that's the way you're going to be, all I can do is pour out more lubricant and at least try to minimize the damage," and the swelling increases. You've still got that fragment wedged in there, and now the meniscus is starting to atrophy because you keep grinding away at it. At the same time the fragment is starting to wear a groove in the bone surface, setting the stage for an arthritic condition, an inflammation, or effusion of the joint.

Pain is now more diffuse and you can't put your finger on the source. (Of course by now it's so tender you probably don't want to touch it anyway.) The muscles controlling the knee attempt to protect the injury by going into spasm and preventing the normal arc of movement. Unable to move through their natural range, the muscles start to atrophy. So now you've got muscle weakness, a locked knee that probably gives way with increasing frequency, swelling of the knee, more pain than you care to think about, you're starting to scratch and damage the surface of the joint, and somewhere, from deep inside, comes an inclination to call a doctor.

Perhaps half of the pain of a traumatic injury is due to accompanying muscle spasms. In a spasm the muscles surrounding the injured part vigorously contract and hold that position—sometimes for days. While such spasms are intensely painful, they're actually the body's way of protecting itself from further injury. Think of it as a built-in splint, immobilizing the damaged part much like a cast immobilizes a broken leg.

Too often, pain is ignored or blunted with medication. This is an invitation to reinjury or even greater injury. When it comes to pain, the individual who self-medicates has a fool for a doctor. If pain persists after two days of self-medication, see your doctor.

5
What's Up, Doc?
Chronic Knee Problems

The majority of people do not suffer from one inglorious moment, but rather develop problems over time and then wonder why their knee is so angry. This type of injury is called chronic—it takes a long time to develop, and once it's around, it's hard to get it to leave.

Here's a collection of conditions, a summary of symptoms and treatment, and a look at the general prognosis.

CHONDROMALACIA PATELLA ("Runner's Knee")

The most common knee complaint is kneecap pain and the most common cause is deterioration of the cartilage on the undersurface of the kneecap. The deterioration is called chondromalacia, the kneecap is the patella, hence the mouthful chondromalacia patella. According to the latest figures (1980), this condition is diagnosed twice as often in women as it is in men; however, in athletes in general, it appears to affect men and women equally.

It is often associated with running and aerobics. Individuals whose feet pronate, or tend to roll toward the inside, are more susceptible to this condition. Dancers and weight lifters are at greater risk due to the number of deep knee bends they perform. Occasionally this condition is caused by some other problem, such as *rheumatoid arthritis,* recurrent bleeding into the knee, or infection. It may also be associated with long-forgotten knee injury. For example, a severe blow to the kneecap—or several over the course of time—may years later creep up on you as chondromalacia. And if you have ever sustained a knee injury requiring repeated cortisone injections or prolonged immobilization, this, too, may predispose you to this degenerative process.

The onset of chondromalacia patella is insidious, progressing slowly and often involving both knees. The exception, of course, is when it's associated with injury to just one knee, such as in an automobile accident with the front of the knee striking the dashboard. If you find yourself victim to this disease, it is not to be ignored. Chondromalacia can lead to degenerative arthritis.

Symptoms

Typically this condition affects an otherwise healthy young person between the ages of twelve and thirty-five who complains of a poorly localized, dull aching pain on the front of the knee. The first pain is likely to result from activity such as running or hiking or after prolonged sitting, such as a long car or plane trip. The symptoms can be aggravated by climbing, walking inclines, or running hills. A crackling sound or grating feeling also often accompanies this problem, but it should be noted that to at least some degree this particular symptom is common in people over the age of twenty.

When your knee is straightened the kneecap is quite mobile, almost "floating." However, when your leg is bent (flexed), the patella sits tightly in its groove. If the kneecap starts to soften around the edges, there are nerve endings that can't take the pressure like they used to and eventually they let you know they are not pleased. So after sitting in one position for a while the classic "theater sign" occurs: Your legs take on a mind of their own and say, "Hey, dummy! Either stand up and stretch or at least grab an aisle seat." Either way, you'll take the pressure off your patella and it will feel better.

Treatment

If your complaints are mild, rest and avoidance of those activities that cause pain are best. This means no kneeling, extensive stair climbing, or prolonged sitting. When you do sit, stretch your legs or put your feet up and relax. Aspirin, or some other non-steroidal anti-inflammatory medication, three to four times a day for a couple of weeks may bring some relief. Warm soaks are also recommended.

Braces can be helpful when symptoms are related to specific activities. The best braces for chondromalacia consist of an elastic sleeve with a central opening for the kneecap and a pad that helps hold the patella in place. There are braces that have pads that totally surround the kneecap. These, however, should be avoided since they can actually hold the kneecap down in the flexed position even during activity. If symptoms are severe, crutches can be used until the pain subsides.

Isometric exercises for the *quadriceps* may also be started, but if they irritate the knee, back off. Don't quit, just back off. Exercising improves quads strength, which will improve patellar tracking and reduce pain. Although you may worry about exercising while in pain, as long as your leg is straight during exercise, pain should be limited. However, exercises that have the knee going through its full range of motion (isotonic exercises) should be avoided, as should squatting. (You'll find appropriate progressive resistance exercises to help you overcome chondromalacia patella in Appendix A.)

If you have chondromalacia, the *worst* exercises are full deep squats, leg presses, "hack squats," and lunges. Jumping activities, such as basketball and volleyball, are also not advised. Runners who suffer from chondromalacia need to take it easy during their recovery, but jogging (on *flat* land) is not considered as stressful as deep squatting or jumping.

If medical management has failed, you may have to consider surgical treatment. There are certain realignment measures that can be done arthroscopically; these will take pressure off of sensitive areas. Arthroscopic shaving is another alternative. In this procedure loose fibers of cartilage are removed, which decreases some of the breakdown products that may cause inflammation. Operative results in general, however, have really been too inconsistent to recommend surgery as an early approach.

So conservative management is preferred. If you can achieve your ideal weight range, avoid activities that involve repetitive squatting or kneeling, and rebuild thigh muscles to normal strength, probably 85 percent of symptoms can be brought under control. That does not mean complete freedom of symptoms, but it does mean results that are as good or even better than currently attainable by surgery.

CHONDROMALACIA PATELLA

Common Name	Who Gets It	Where It Hurts
Runner's Knee	Runners Aerobic dancers The overweight (may be secondary to subluxating patella) May follow traumatic injury ("dashboard knee")	The kneecap

Other Symptoms	What to Do	Often Confused With
All bent-knee activities cause discomfort	Avoid bent-knee activities	Tear of the medial meniscus
Grinding, occasional swelling, sensation of locking Weakness Knee fatigues quickly	Strengthening leg muscles is critical Orthotics may be beneficial. Use cold packs and anti-inflammatory medication.	

PATELLA SUBLUXATION (Dislocated Kneecap)

The knee joint is created by the end of the thighbone (femur) sitting snugly on top of the shinbone (tibia). Near the end of the femur there is a track that holds the kneecap as it protects the joint. At times the kneecap can be knocked completely off the groove; technically, this is a dislocated kneecap. At other times the kneecap may be "riding" on the edge and not completely dislocated; this is when we say the patella has subluxated.

Sometimes individuals have a congenital defect and the kneecap tends to run off the track or "subluxate" in the face of a severe sudden twist or constant stress. Picture a sliding door with a tendency to run off the track momentarily because it wasn't built right. For other people there may not be anything inherently wrong with the knee; a traumatic event, such as a fall, dislocates the kneecap and the next time it takes less trauma to cause a recurrence.

This is probably the second most common disorder of the kneecap. It is also one that has captured the imagination of many orthopedic specialists. For example, by 1959 there were at least 137 surgical methods designed to solve this problem. This is a sure sign that no one really knows what will consistently work.

Yet we have to keep trying because this problem comprises a significant segment of knee injuries and represents a major cause of internal derangement. Each time a kneecap dislocates there will likely be cartilage or joint damage, a fracture of the undersurface of the kneecap, or even a fracture of the lateral femoral *condyle,* which is the bone end that the kneecap slides over as it dislocates. If that's not bad enough, over time this condition can lead to the onset of arthritis and further degenerative damage.

Symptoms

Because the subluxation happens quickly, the patient rarely re-

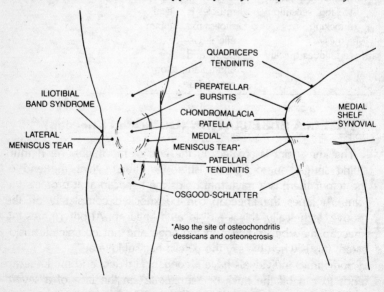

The sites of major knee problems

ports a completely dislocated kneecap. Instead, the complaint is generally of poorly localized knee pain and a history of vague complaints that the knee "gives way," "pops," "locks," or "goes out of place." In fact, what generally convinces someone to seek medical advice is not the pain of subluxation but rather the pain caused by the degenerative changes taking place inside the knee.

The pain is aggravated by both activity, especially stair climbing, and inactivity with the knee bent (such as in an automobile or theater). During sports participation, subluxation occurs when your knee gives way when you turn, cut back, or push off during activity.

Typically, the first dislocation is recalled with great clarity: "I slid into second base, I hit the baseman, and 'Pow!'—I thought my knee was coming off!" The next dislocation was almost as painful, but the third time not nearly so. After that the kneecap goes off its track and there's a moment of instability and that's about it. There's little pain and hardly any swelling.

That first episode causes everything anchoring the kneecap to become stretched or torn. The muscles and tendons heal, but in a lengthened position, and after a while they become very stretched out. The longer the problem is ignored, the greater degenerative problem there will be to manage.

The complaints—locking, giving way, pain, and swelling—are the same symptoms associated with meniscal injuries, which means diagnosis can be difficult. I've seen people who have had their meniscus removed when in fact their problem was really a subluxating patella. This obviously didn't solve the problem and often resulted in severe arthritic degeneration as the subluxation continued.

One of the key diagnostic features of this problem is something called the "apprehension sign." People with subluxation often display marked apprehension when the doctor moves to push the patella laterally while testing for stability or increased mobility. This isn't as sadistic as it sounds. A good examiner will note this apprehension and back off, hoping to avoid the "throat sign," which is where the patient grabs the examiner if he goes one step further.

Treatment

The most notable feature of patella subluxation is a wasting of the vastus medialus muscles, which are part of the quadriceps. The quads hold the patella tightly against the femur, so returning these muscles to peak condition is a primary goal of treatment. Nonpainful leg lifts and leg lifts with weights are important in getting the kneecap back on track. Support by bracing is also often recommended.

Studies suggest that with conservative treatment—that is, nonsurgical remedies—dislocations become less frequent over time and there is little evidence of osteoarthritis. For people who have undergone surgery there is a higher recurrence rate, a risk that further surgery may be necessary, and a disturbingly high incidence of osteoarthritis. Therefore, surgery should be considered only after conservative rehabilitative techniques have failed.

PATELLA SUBLUXATION

Common Name	Who Gets It	Where It Hurts
Dislocated kneecap	Females slightly more than males Players of contact sports	Kneecap

Other Symptoms	What to Do	Often Confused With
Swelling Limited movement A feeling the knee may collapse	Strengthen muscles Stretch hamstrings Use braces, knee supports, possibly orthotics	Chondromalacia patella Tears of the medial meniscus

BURSITIS ("Housemaid's Knee")

The letters -*itis* mean inflammation, so bursitis is inflammation of the bursa. The what? The bursa are little empty sacs around any joint that for the most part go unnoticed—until they fill with fluid and swell. They're a little like air bags in cars, tucked away, out of sight and out of mind until—WHAM!—and they're suddenly real hard to ignore.

There are fourteen bursas around the knee and any one of them can become inflamed. What generally happens is that something irritates the knee, maybe the knee strikes a sharp object, or maybe the knee's owner has been kneeling a bit too much, and the bursa decides the knee could do with some extra protection. So it fills with fluid or blood and tries to protect the knee from further injury.

That's great for the knee but, if it's your knee, you will find there's a cost for this added protection: intense pain.

The bursa in front of the knee is what gets irritated by too much kneeling and the result is a bursitis known as "housemaid's knee." Of course you don't have to be anywhere near a kitchen floor to have angry bursa; carpenters, bricklayers, plumbers, and even ministers are often victims.

If you have gout, gouty crystals may form in the knee causing irritation and bursitis.

Symptoms

Localized pain, swelling, and tenderness are the hallmarks of bursitis.

Treatment

The first order of business is to eliminate the irritant. For example, either get a long-handled mop or pray standing up. Then oral anti-inflammatory drugs will help calm the bursa. In severe cases the bursa may have to be drained, the area injected with cortisone, and the fluid checked for special conditions like gout or infection. One to three injections of cortisone generally brings quick relief.

Bursitis is usually a very self-limiting phenomenon, unless it is also associated with gout, or arthritis, or some other condition that will cause continued irritation and continually angry bursa.

BURSITIS		
Common Name	**Who Gets It**	**Where It Hurts**
Housemaid's Knee	Kneelers (carpenters, plumbers, brick-layers	Front of the knee is most common
Other Symptoms	**What to Do**	**Often Confused With**
Swelling Limited movement	Ice/friction massage Anti-inflammatories Protective pads	Chondromalacia patella

PATELLAR TENDINITIS ("Jumper's Knee")

The kneecap is connected to the front thigh muscle and shinbone by patellar and quadriceps tendons. A small tear here causes tendinitis, or "jumper's knee." This condition is usually sport-related, represents overuse of the involved tendon, and is common among basketball and volleyball players, hurdlers, and dancers. It may also be a complicating factor of Osgood-Schlatter disease in children (Chapter 26).

Symptoms

A sharp pain in and around the patella is usually exacerbated by jumping. The knee may show swelling, redness, even warmth around the kneecap. Straight leg raising also causes pain.

Various stages have been classically described: Stage 1—aching after participation; Stage 2—aching during participation; Stage 3—aching and pain during participation, which is now affecting ability to participate; Stage 4—the catastrophic event that is caused by deterioration of the tendon to the point that it ruptures. Ouch!

Treatment

Jumping must be avoided for one to three weeks until the pain stops. Anti-inflammatory agents and massage can be helpful. In ice/friction massage, ice is rubbed on the skin for several minutes until numbness occurs. (Ice is also used with cross-fiber friction massage, followed by the use of a dry washcloth to rewarm the skin. This is repeated twice, ending with ice to stimulate the circulation.)

For some people, shoe orthotics, knee wraps, or a "jumper's knee brace" may be beneficial.

As with chondromalacia patellae, quadriceps-strengthening and -stretching exercises can prevent recurrence.

My own experience suggests that about 70 percent of patients seem to be able to arrest their condition at the Stage 1 level with braces, an exercise program, use of minimal anti-inflammatory medication, and ice/friction massage. Of the remaining 30 percent, two out of three end up with more aggressive medical management, including perhaps a steroid injection, a more prolonged period of rest and recovery, and, in truly severe cases, perhaps surgery. And 10 percent will have to significantly modify their activities and go to a different sport. For example, basketball or volleyball will have to be replaced with a less knee-demanding activity.

Strangely enough, this problem was much more common several years ago than it is now. Although there's no concrete proof, I would like to ascribe this to better training habits, improved training surfaces, better shoes, and better exercise regimens.

PATELLAR TENDINITIS		
Common Name	**Who Gets It**	**Where It Hurts**
Jumper's knee	High jumpers Hurdlers Dancers Volleyball players Basketball players	Front of the knee
Other Symptoms	**What to Do**	**Often Confused With**
Swelling Redness Warmth	Ice/friction massage Anti-inflammatories Decrease jumping Strengthen muscles Elastic knee supports	Chondromalacia patella

ILIOTIBIAL BAND FRICTION SYNDROME

The tendinitis associated with runners and dancers is called iliotibial band friction syndrome (IBFS); it involves a tendon that runs from the hip down to the outer (lateral) side of the knee. As the knee flexes and extends, the iliotibial band rubs against the end of the thighbone (femur), which ends in two elliptical notches called condyles. (Picture a dog's bone. The rounded endpoints are condyles.) Excessive motion or tightness of the tendon can produce irritation when it rubs against the outer condyle. Because this is an especially common problem among runners, you'll find considerable more detail in Chapter 19.

Symptoms

The first indication of IBFS will likely be a post-aerobic burning pain. It is a very specific pain that occurs at the end of your thighbone at a point known as the lateral femoral condyle. Soon it occurs during your aerobic activity and eventually prevents or limits your activity or, at the very least, limits your time due to pain. For example, the pain may become so severe that it is impossible to run more than a short distance, which may be only a fraction of your usual mileage. Sports such as squash or tennis may also produce discomfort, as will repetitive *flexion-extension* movements such as cycling, skiing, or weight lifting.

With running, IBFS is often associated with a rapid increase in mileage, a course that involves hills, or a running surface that is at a slight angle.

Treatment

Initial treatment may include ice/friction massage and stretching of the iliotibial band. For specific stretching exercises see Appendix A.

Anti-inflammatory medication, such as aspirin, speeds recovery, and if, after three weeks, the pain is still persistent, a hydrocortisone injection may be helpful while you continue to limit activity, perform stretching exercises, and change your individual activities to prevent recurrence. The latter may involve moving your activity to a softer surface, rerouting to avoid downhill or sidehill running, and varying mileage patterns (alternating short distances with long).

A shoe insert or orthotic may also be beneficial if there is a mild malalignment of the knee or ankle.

ILIOTIBIAL BAND FRICTION SYNDROME

Common Name	Who Gets It	Where It Hurts
None	Runners Dancers Bicylists Men more than women	Outer side of the knee

Other Symptoms	What to Do	Often Confused With
Swelling Pain after running a specific distance (one-half to 10 miles)	Strengthen muscles Ice/friction massage Change running surface Proper footwear Correct form	Tear of the lateral meniscus Stress fractures

PATHOLOGICAL SYNOVIAL PLICAE

The diagnosis of pathological synovial plicae is over-applied and over-discussed. Yes, it does exist, but it doesn't deserve near the attention it has received.

Plicae were once considered a harmless developmental anomaly; today they are called by some authorities "the great imitators." These are developmental leftovers that exist in anywhere from 18 to 60 percent of normal knees, depending on the medical authority who is reporting them and his or her care in detecting these folds of the knee lining. In order to understand this problem you must know a little about how the knee develops in a human body. By the eighth week of development the knee is formed of three synovial compartments, which are separated by thin, membranous walls. During the fourth fetal month these walls are usually reabsorbed back into the body, leaving the three compartments fused into one knee. However, sometimes these walls, or some portion of them, remain. These fetal remnants are called plicae.

Prior to the advent of the arthroscope, no one paid much attention to these remnants, which were considered incapable of causing any problems. They were an annoyance to the surgeon who sometimes had to get his equipment through toughened plica tissue, but for the most part they appeared to be a pretty insignificant knee structure. Then surgeons began reporting that in some painful knees the only internal problem they could find were the fibrous bands of tissue, and when these bands were divided the pain was relieved. Eventually physicians began to recognize these structures as capable of causing acute and chronic knee pain.

Trauma can injure the plicae, producing inflammation. This may be a simple stretch, tear, or contusion, but when the body repairs the injury the fold has lost some of its elasticity and becomes more fibrous and abrasive. Activity only increases the irritation and minor trauma increases the abnormal thickening of the once pliant tissue. Eventually pain may develop with activity or a single traumatic event may cause a knee-jerk response and plenty of pain.

Symptoms

Although the incidence of plicae in the general population may be quite high, only 15 to 20 percent are ever responsible for symptoms. The most common complaints include tenderness or aching pain, over the condyles or above the kneecap, that worsens with activity. There may also be swelling or a feeling of "tightness" in the knee, weakness or instability in the knee, and sound effects such as popping, snapping, or clicking. It is rare, however, to find a patient who is fully disabled by the symptoms and incapable of pursuing either work or school activities. Individuals with this condition generally do not have pain when standing still.

Pain is increased with repetitive activities, such as running and jumping, and is commonly aggravated by a quadriceps-strengthening program, but it will subside with rest.

Here, too, the diagnosis is typically one of exclusion. Frequently the symptoms suggest either chondromalacia patella, a meniscal tear, or a number of other internal derangements of the knee. These possibilities must be carefully ruled out before concluding that a plica is the sole cause of pain.

Treatment

If your screaming plicae have resulted from overuse, you have at least an 80 percent chance of responding well to conservative measures consisting of rest, ice initially and then heat, and keeping your legs extended while sitting. Medication, such as aspirin, may be beneficial, as are hamstring- and quadriceps-stretching exercises. If your symptoms followed blunt trauma, such as a fall or the striking of a solid object, or a twisting injury, the prospects are pretty much reversed: Your chance of relief by conservative measures is 20 percent or less. Fortunately, 90 percent of patients undergoing arthroscopic removal of these folds report good or excellent results. Complications are rare and recovery quick. So if, after three to four months, symptomatic plicae have failed to respond to conservative measures, it's probably time to consider anthroscopy.

PATHOLOGICAL SYNOVIAL PLICAE

Common Name	Who Gets It	Where It Hurts
None	Knee injured (from striking an object)	Inner (medial) side

Other Symptoms	What to Do	Often Confused With
Swelling	Strengthen muscles	Tear of the medial
Pseudo-locking	Ice/friction massage	meniscus
Clicking	Avoid squatting and kneeling	Chondromalacia patella
	Anti-inflammatories	

SPONTANEOUS OSTEONECROSIS

In separate chapters we'll discuss arthritis. Whereas arthritis is a gradual degenerative condition, which develops over months or years, spontaneous osteonecrosis has sometimes been described by patients as "instant arthritis." It is a more common problem for older individuals, with the average patient about sixty-five years old, although the range is from forty to eighty-five. We really don't know what causes this condition, but its typical presentation is a real attention-getter.

Symptoms

A sudden, severe pain, rarely associated with trauma of any sort, occurs spontaneously. If you've experienced this pain, you probably remember exactly what you were doing when the pain struck. The pain most often occurs on the inner side of the knee. It is not improved by rest, and weight-bearing activities, such as walking, may aggravate the pain. It does not subside with time. During this early phase the knee appears "locked" because it's prevented from complete extension or flexion due to pain, effusion, and muscle spasm. It's not a true "locked" knee because there is no mechanical block, although a mechanical block does sometimes develop.

The future isn't bright for those knees struck with spontaneous osteonecrosis. Although for a few lucky people the pain will subside in three to six months, others will continue to experience degenerative changes within their knee, causing pain and a limiting of function. This may occur rapidly, although the typical case develops slowly. The prognosis is sometimes dramatically poor and rarely good.

During the first four to eight weeks X rays are normal, then sometime between two and six months changes are often noted by X rays.

Treatment

If diagnosed early, pain medication is best, along with crutches or a cane and at least six months of isometric quadriceps exercises. Although the threat of continued arthritic-type changes is great, the majority of patients seem to respond to this conservative approach.

Unfortunately, S.O. victims sometimes show (in X rays) a lesion actually creating a growing crater along the inner ends of the femur and tibia. If major problems persist and there is increasing deformity one to three years following the onset of symptoms, surgery, ranging from arthroscopy to a total knee replacement, may be necessary. The best success, in chronic cases, is seen with a high tibial osteotomy. That may sound like a religious ceremony, but what it means is that by removing a wedge of bone on the lateral, or outer, side of the knee, the knee undergoes a realignment. This has the same effect as realigning a car's tires: It corrects the alignment problem caused by the lesion and takes the load off of the injured bone by transferring it to another part of the knee.

SPONTANEOUS OSTEONECROSIS

Common Name	Who Gets It	Where It Hurts
None	Older people	Inner (medial) side of the knee

Other Symptoms	What to Do	Often Confused With
Swelling Locking Loss of movement	External support (cane or crutches) Limit activity Strengthen muscles	Medial meniscal tear

6

What's Up, Doc? (Revisited)
Acute Knee Problems

So you've finally found time to go out and shoot some baskets—
first exercise in a week—and what happens but your knee gives
way just when you plant and pivot, about to drive in with your killer
slam dunk. What's wrong? If it's acute, you should find an answer
in this chapter.

ACUTE MENISCAL TEARS (see also "Sprains," this chapter)

We've already talked a little about the knee's shock absorbers,
the menisci. When you talk of a torn cartilage it's the meniscus that
has been folded, spindled, and . . . well, you know.

Acute tears most commonly occur from a twisting action while
putting weight on the knee; you may feel a tearing sensation at the
time of injury. Repetitive squatting or kneeling as well as natural
aging processes can weaken the menisci and set the stage for an
acute meniscal injury. In fact, it's amazing how little force is necessary to damage even a healthy meniscus: simply squatting to pick
up something from the floor or getting out of a car can be the last
straw that completes the tear. Of course not all cartilage is created
equal. God gave some people top-of-the-line cushioning while others got brand X.

Symptoms

When a meniscus is first torn, bleeding within the joint irritates the lining, or synovium, of the knee. In an attempt to wash away the irritant, the knee increases its production of synovial fluid and the knee swells.

One of the most common tears of the meniscus is the "bucket-handle" tear. The meniscus develops a split and part of it becomes trapped within the joint. When this portion of meniscus is separated, yet still attached at either end, it appears to be the shape of a bucket, with the entrapped portion representing the handle. The knee is locked and prevents complete leg straightening. There's also pain along the edge of the "bucket" and swelling, usually two to six hours post-injury.

Often you try to ignore a damaged meniscus and, for a time, your knee cooperates. Some movement returns and you begin to think that you're going to recover. Of course your leg won't straighten completely or bend as far as it used to, but between these extremes there is acceptable movement. However, some swelling simply refuses to go away, so you break down and make an appointment with your doctor.

Diagnosis is often one of exclusion, and unless your knee is locked by a bucket-handle tear, it may be weeks after your initial injury before you know exactly what's wrong with your knee. The most revealing symptoms are tenderness, inability to squat, duck, walk, or bounce up and down while standing. There is also pain when you attempt to rotate with the feet planted.

Treatment

A torn meniscus means surgery most of the time. But today most physicians agree that unless the meniscus is definitely unstable or symptomatic, it should be left in—or only part of it removed—to protect the knee from osteoarthritis. That's why 90 percent of the nearly 100,000 meniscectomies done in the United States today are only partial meniscectomies.

Certain tears in the meniscus can be sutured. However, this is not always possible, and it does involve an extended period of disability and recovery. There are particular modifying factors that affect a decision to do a meniscal repair. First, what is the complexity of the tear? It is much harder to get multiple tears to heal than it is if there is one discreet tear. Second, where has the tear(s) occurred? The outer one third of the meniscus has an excellent blood supply, which means it has the greatest capacity for healing. There are individual variations, but in general the farther into the meniscus a tear occurs, the less chance there is of healing and recovery.

Other considerations include the age of the injured, and his or her individual healing potential and life-style. Usually the younger person is the most amenable technically and socially to the repair process. For a meniscectomy, you're on crutches for a few days; for a meniscal repair, six to eight weeks. If a simple, partial meniscectomy is performed, recovery takes about six weeks. For a meniscal repair, recovery will take six to twelve months. That's a big difference. I don't think it makes sense to try a repair on a sixty-year-old construction worker who is moving, twisting, and squatting all day as a part of his job. Will he be willing, let alone able, to take a year off or a reassignment in order to recover from the more complicated surgery? On the other hand, a total meniscectomy on a patient under the age of sixteen can be a real catastrophe. Ten to fifteen years later that individual may face real arthritic problems. So if I tore my meniscus, I'd say just take it out arthroscopically. If my daughter tore hers, I would want it repaired if possible. If there were multiple tears, I'd need to see some statistics to indicate that the repair will heal and she will be better off after a year of recovery.

Exercise

A large meniscal tear that causes the knee to lock, block, or give way probably will not be affected by a strengthening program. Even so, a rehabilitation program is valuable; if surgery is performed, the strengthening program will help prevent further injury and facilitate postoperative recovery. Whenever a knee injury occurs, muscle strength, power, and endurance quickly weaken in the affected leg. A loss of just 15 to 20 percent of muscle strength significantly increases the risk of reinjury. During the first two weeks most people will have at least 15 percent deficiency, and by the time I see most of my patients, one month after the onset of symptoms the vast majority have lost 30 to 40 percent of their muscle strength.

MENISCAL TEARS

Common Name	Who Gets It	Where It Hurts
Torn cartilage	Players of contact sports (esp. football, soccer)	Localized pain
	Skiers, older people, carpenters, plumbers, construction workers	

Other symptoms	What to Do	Often Confused With
Swelling	Arthroscopic removal	Torn ligaments
Locked knee	of the torn portion	
Tearing sensation	of the meniscus	
Pain with rotation of the knee		

DEGENERATIVE MENISCAL TEARS

The meniscal tear most often associated with aging is called a cleavage-type tear. This may sound sexy, but the pain and swelling associated with the horizontal separation is hardly alluring. (To get an idea of this separation, picture the venetian-blind effect that occurs when a favorite pair of blue jeans wears out at the knee.)

Often the problem can be brought under control with exercises that build power and endurance in the quadriceps and hamstrings. (See Appendix A.) That assumes, however, that you avoid the repetitive squatting or kneeling that most likely caused the problem. Otherwise, arthroscopy can be performed and the torn portion of the meniscus can be removed.

LIGAMENT TEARS ("Sprained Knee")

We've discussed how the ligaments act as the scaffolding for the bones of the knee. The collateral ligaments run up the inside and outside of the knee, while the anterior cruciate ligament and the posterior cruciate ligament cross within the joint. A sprain occurs when any of these ligaments are stretched excessively or torn.

The inner or medial collaterial ligament (MCL) is the most common site of knee sprains. Indeed, the MCL is probably 50 times more likely to be injured than the ACL. (Fortunately, most MCL injuries are of such a minor nature that they are never even called to a doctor's attention.) The ACL is often torn in contact sports. To give you an idea of the scope of knee sprains, by conservative estimate at least 50,000 occur each year in the United States just among skiers. Fortunately, less than 15 percent require surgery.

Symptoms

The Standard Nomenclature of Athletic Injuries, published by the American Medical Association (impressive, huh), defines three categories of ligamentous injury:

1. *Grade 1* "mild" sprains are those with mild tenderness, minimal hemorrhage and swelling, no abnormal motion, and minimal disability. There are minor tears of ligament fibers. There is minimal loss of strength, no lengthening, and no loss of function.

2. *Grade 2* "moderate" sprains are those with moderate loss of function, more joint reaction (i.e., swelling and tenderness), slight to moderate abnormal motion, and partial tearing of ligamentous tissues. There is stretching of some ligament fibers and tearing of some.

3. *Grade 3* "severe" sprains are those with marked abnormal motion, indicating a complete tear of the ligament. This causes a total loss of strength and functional capacity and may require surgical repair.

Treatment

Back in the 1950s, casting was the primary treatment for an MCL injury. (Back then ACL injuries were basically ignored!) Then we went through a phase when surgery was the "treatment" of choice. As a matter of fact, during the seventies MCL repair was the most common knee ligament surgery. However, during the last few years there has been an astronomical drop in the incidence of MCL surgical repairs. What we learned is that Grade 1 and Grade 2 MCL sprains will heal just as well with conservative treatment as they will with surgical intervention. So surgery is now generally reserved for only the most serious, Grade 3, MCL injuries.

In general the treatment for sprains depends on the severity of the injury. For a mild sprain, RICE is advised: rest, ice, compression, and elevation. Usually there is a relatively quick return to activity. Two to three weeks is not uncommon, although we'll soon explain why the recovery period may be even longer.

If it is a second-degree sprain, the treatment will vary depending on the functional requirements of the individual, the pain and discomfort being experienced, and how badly other knee structures, such as cartilage or muscles, have been damaged. Also, one ligament may have a second-degree injury while another might have suffered a more severe third-degree injury, so strains are often far from cut-and-dried phenomenon.

The knee will need protection for one to six weeks in the form of a removable splint and an intermittent range of motion exercises or a brace that allows for limited movement.

For the most severe (Grade 3) sprains, surgical repair is often considered, with prolonged (three to eight weeks) splint or brace protection generally recommended. Some continued protection may even be appropriate beyond eight weeks. It should be noted that the bracing is not meant to simply provide stability; the surgical repair should do that. Instead, it is to protect and prevent reinjury while allowing for the healing of the ligament.

Perhaps the biggest problem in treating sprains is undertreating mild ones and overtreating the moderate and severe ones. Many mild sprains are functioning again within two to three weeks, yet by definition a Grade 1 sprain has damaged tissue and is weakened for a longer period of time, perhaps several months. The real hazard with Grade 1 sprains is that you will not fully appreciate your injury and you will return to activity too soon and find yourself reinjured. Unfortunately, when this happens the resulting sprain may be much more serious than the original.

While it may take only a few weeks to return to action following a sprain, actual healing may take up to two years. During the first year you will reach a significant plateau of healing and then slow healing will likely continue for another year.

Surgical Repair

Since ligaments do not have a rich blood supply, it should be remembered that they do not heal well. They should be evaluated for possible repair. Well, they can be ignored, but that does engender a certain amount of risk and a definite degree of suspense: When will your trick knee go into its next act?

If you and your doctor decide that surgical repair is necessary, the particular approach will depend on your precise injury. For a severe MCL injury, there needs to be some open surgery since the ligament is not accessible to our arthroscopes. (You'll read more about arthroscopy later when we detail the advantages of this technology.)

Although the ACL is accessible to our microscopic surgical tools, this ligament is much more difficult to repair. The greatest likelihood for a successful repair occurs when a piece of either the femur or tibia actually breaks off with the ACL attached. That happens when the bone gives way before all of the forces can be transmitted to the ligament. It's easier to repair a bone than it is a torn ligament, unfortunately.

Most surgeons believe that when the ACL is torn from the bone at either end, it should be reattached, since the chances of normal function after repair are good. Toward this end, orthopedists have developed a number of suturing and stapling techniques. Sadly, despite the initial enthusiasm, we're finding that many patients undergoing this type of ACL repair really aren't healing well. When we have had an opportunity to look at some of these patients later, what we find is pretty worthless scar tissue instead of good resilient tissue surrounding all that fancy medical handiwork.

Still, even this limited success is better than what we see if the anterior cruciate ligament has been torn interstitially, that is, along the ligament itself as opposed to a break at the point it connects to bone. Although a tear occurs at only one point along the ligament, there is failure all along the ligament before it ruptures. To the eye it appears to be intact, but microscopically there is noticeable damage up and down the ligament. It's comparable to what you might have experienced if you've ever broken a rubber band, tied it back together with a knot, only to have it snap apart again an inch away from the original break. It looked fine, but what you couldn't see was that in the constant stretching of the rubber band it lost its normal elasticity, its continuity, and even though only one small part broke, the rest of it was severely weakened. That's what happens in most ACL tears.

ACL Reconstruction

For these and other reasons, reconstruction is becoming more popular than repair: Other tissue or synthetic material is used to graft or reconstruct the ligament. If possible, someone's own tissue is preferable to any of the artificial ligaments that are available at this time. (This technology is discussed in great detail in the epilogue.) Rather than repair the torn ACL, a tendon alongside the knee is moved over and down as a replacement. The process may include looping the tendon to actually provide more strength than the original. Some of the patients who have had this surgery were professional or college athletes who had been sidelined by continuing instability following previous surgery. Many were restored to their former levels of performance.

Several popular operations use the patellar tendon to replace the ACL because it's one of the strongest grafts available. A potential problem with this approach is that the patellar tendon is a vital structure and taking one third to one half of it to do the reconstruction strikes me as robbing Peter to pay Paul. The penalty is often extra wear of the kneecap and difficulty in regaining flexion at the knee.

Non-Surgical Management of the Torn ACL

All of this assumes that you and your doctor decided on a surgical approach. Within the last few years we have come to realize that, contrary to earlier belief, a torn ACL is not necessarily the beginning of the end. Although a complete solution to the torn anterior cruciate ligament has yet to be devised, numerous options are available. And, indeed, one of those options is to learn how to live with it. Probably at least 60 percent or more of all patients can tolerate loss of this ligament. It depends on the amount of laxity present and the desired level of activity.

Age is also a factor. Ninety percent of the people undergoing ACL repairs or reconstruction are between nineteen and twenty-seven years old. The older person probably is not going to place the demand on their knee that someone younger will. And a torn ACL usually implies modification of life-style, including both athletic and vocational endeavors.

For example, living with a torn anterior cruciate ligament probably means living without running-and-cutting sports such as basketball and racquetball. Any activity involving sudden stops and turns
would simply be harder to take and much more hazardous. Climbing or working on rough terrain or slippery surfaces would also be
ill-advised. Remember, the cruciate ligaments prevent the bones
from slipping backward or forward out of joint. Without an ACL for
added support, going down hills or stepping in a hole can be a lot
more treacherous because you just don't have the resiliency and
protection you once had. This means you can still run after your
bus if you have a clear path, but stepping off the curb could send
you to the ground.

In our office we're currently studying the natural histories of
patients who had untreated but documented anterior cruciate ligament tears. About 80 percent of them are satisfied, but we are
going to find out what they had to change in order to accommodate
their knee condition.

TORN LIGAMENTS

Common Name	Who Gets It	Where It Hurts
Sprain	Players of contact sports (esp. bas- ketball, football) Skiers Victims of falls or accidents	Localized in Grades 1 and 2 Diffuse in Grade 3

Other Symptoms	What to Do	Often Confused With
Swelling Instability Loss of motion Rehabilitation program	Immobilize (brace or crutches) Ice or cold packs	Fractures Dislocated patella

"THE TERRIBLE TRIAD"

Of all the possible traumatic injuries, there is one that is a four-
star pain in the knee. A player whose foot is planted receives a blow
to the outside of the joint, forcing the large bones inward. This puts

an extraordinary amount of pressure on internal structures and may stretch or tear the meniscus when it is crushed between the bones; the anterior cruciate ligament may also give way, and the medical collateral ligament also stretches or tears. This orthopedic nightmare is called *"the terrible triad."*

Treatment

Due to the magnitude of the injury, 90 percent of the time this means surgery, and generally not a simple arthroscopic procedure but a combination of open and arthroscopic surgery. Recovery for ligamentous injuries in general ranges from nine to eighteen months and in the case mentioned above we're probably talking about the high end of that range. Someone who has suffered the terrible triad has actually suffered two traumas: an injury trauma and a surgical trauma. It is big surgery to put it all back together. A lot of tissue must be cut through to work on the areas affected. All of that has to heal while the person undergoes all types of muscular rehabilitation.

The prognosis is pretty good, however. In my experience 85 percent of all patients report good or excellent results postoperatively. Only 5 percent report fair results, and 10 percent say their condition is unsatisfactory.

FRACTURES

There are two types of fractures affecting athletes: traumatic and stress. Major trauma, such as a fall down a flight of stairs or a car accident, often causes a fracture. One traumatic blow in sports, which could be the indelicate landing of a 250-pound tackle or a knee dive into the floor, is all it takes to cause a fracture.

A sheer force crashing into the kneecap can knock a piece of bone off of the patella or the patella track. A direct blow can crack or damage the kneecap's surface or it can force the patella back into its groove and fracture the backside of the patella.

The other type of fracture, a stress fracture, may comprise as much as 10 percent of all sports injuries and up to 16 percent of all injuries to runners. A stress fracture is the result of repeated stress from excessive motion or impact shock. The result is a series of microscopic cracks that, over time, become larger and larger until eventually symptoms develop. Because the symptoms are similar to a number of other conditions, the first diagnosis is often wrong. The most common misdiagnosis is probably tendinitis, with bursitis and "runner's knee" also getting a share of blame. If your knee doesn't respond to therapy within a couple of weeks, a physician will usually become suspicious and order further tests, hoping to find evidence of a stress fracture. Thus, stress fractures are often a diagnosis of exclusion, which means the examining physician first figures out what is *not* causing the pain and then proceeds toward a diagnosis of stress fracture.

Don't be too hard on your doctor if he or she first misses a stress fracture. Besides the fact that the symptoms echo a number of other complaints, another confounder is that symptoms may precede X-ray evidence by up to three months and, in a significant number of stress fractures, there may never be positive X-ray evidence at all. Fortunately, conventional X rays may be supplemented by a bone scan (radionuclide bone scintigraphy) if there is a high suspicion of stress fracture. This has shown to be a very sensitive diagnostic tool, capable of detecting stress fractures within seventy-two hours of onset of pain. A few facilities are also beginning to use *magnetic resonance imaging* for stress fracture detection.

Symptoms

Bone pain is the primary symptom of fractures. The pain begins mildly and gradually worsens. The longer the stress fracture continues to be stressed and goes untreated, the more severe the pain becomes. Localized tenderness and swelling, as well as pain related to activity, are also common, but again these are hardly specific complaints.

Treatment

For traumatic fractures, the first step of all treatment is to recognize the fracture. It's important that fractures be treated within the first week in order to avoid further injury and to guide healing. Sometimes treatment is limited to immobilization (usually a brace or a cast), rest, and protection. For complicated fractures, surgery may be necessary to do internal repair with pins, wires, screws, and plates in order to hold everything in place during healing.

The patient often returns quickly to day-to-day activities, but recreational activities are severely limited during recovery. Cycling, swimming, and running in water are sometimes permitted as alternative activities to maintain fitness. Stretching and flexibility exercises are emphasized, as well as local muscle strengthening, stretching, and retraining.

Once an individual has been pain-free for ten to fourteen days, there is a gradual reintroduction to sports.

Perhaps the single most important factor in avoiding stress fracture reinjury is a schedule of alternate-day activity. In other words, if you're a runner, your best bet for avoiding stress fractures might be to alternate running with bicycling, or just take a day off between runs. One study reported in *Military Medicine* (147:285–87, 1982), found that such a recovery period during training cut the stress fracture rate in military recruits by one third.

The average time to recovery for traumatic fractures is ten to thirteen weeks. For stress fractures, four to ten weeks is generally required.

FRACTURES—TRAUMATIC

Common Name	Who Gets It	Where It Hurts
Broken bone	Players of contact sports (esp. skiing, football, roller-skating) Victims of falls or accidents	Localized pain

Other Symptoms	What to Do	Often Confused With
Swelling	Immobilize	Dislocated patella
Limited movement	Splinting	Sprains
Throbbing	Crutches	
Warmth	Elevation	
Pain even at rest	Ice	

FRACTURES—STRESS		
Common Name	**Who Gets It**	**Where It Hurts**
Shinsplints	Runners Weight lifters High jumpers	Localized pain
Other Symptoms	**What to Do**	**Often Confused With**
Minimal swelling Pain with activity	Decrease activity Strengthen muscles	Tendinitis Bursitis

7

Arthritis
Is It or Isn't It?

Arthritis is the nation's number one chronic disease, affecting over one in seven Americans, or nearly 41 million people. The most common form of arthritis, osteoarthritis, can be identified in the knees of one third of all persons by the age of thirty and affects nearly everyone by the age of sixty. Although often considered an ailment of the elderly, experts who know better call arthritis everybody's disease. It haunts the athletically active regardless of age and is a real problem for a quarter of a million children under the age of sixteen.

Many individuals have "silent" arthritis, that is, they do not suffer the pain, limitation of motion, joint instability, and deformity that are the hallmarks of this disease. Still, about one third to one half of all people with arthritis have a condition serious enough to consult a doctor about their symptoms. The good news is that only a small percentage of this group have severe pain and disability. The bad news is that many people ignore early symptoms or delay effective countermeasures, thus aggravating the problem and sometimes causing permanent crippling. It may seem ludicrous, but it is true: The average individual with arthritis waits four years after symptoms develop before seeking medical help! By then a lot of damage has already taken place.

WHAT IS ARTHRITIS?

Although the pain of arthritis may be new to you, it's one of the oldest identifiable diseases on earth. While Adam's bones probably began creaking shortly after he took up residence outside of Eden, he was not the disease's first victim. A giant dinosaur named *Diplodocus Longus* holds that honor. Today man's aching joints are joined by those of birds, amphibians, reptiles, and mammals. The animals that are spared tend to have cartilaginous skeletons instead of bony skeletons, which means sharks have never experienced arthritis but porpoises have. So it appears that arthritis developed at the same time that bone did during the course of evolution.

One might expect, with this kind of long-term experience, that we should by now have a clear understanding of this disease, but in fact arthritis is still poorly understood and the source of many misconceptions. Part of the problem is that arthritis is a word that is used to label about 100 conditions that involve aches and pains in joints and connective tissue. The "big three" are osteoarthritis, rheumatoid arthritis, and gout.

Osteoarthritis (OA)

We discussed cartilage earlier and explained how it is a tough, elastic tissue that acts as a shock absorber and keeps the bones from rubbing against each other. In osteoarthritis (OA) there is a gradual wearing away of this cartilage, which leads to discomfort, pain, stiffness, grating, and, sometimes, deformity. The pain is often localized to only one or a few joints. Classically, the pain of OA occurs with movement and is relieved by rest; however, many OA patients will experience some degree of achy pain when they resume activity following a period of rest. Pain may also be worse at the end of the day.

Factors contributing to OA include repetitive stress and injury, heredity, and too much weight. An estimated 30 million Americans suffer from osteoarthritis, with the greatest incidence among the older population.

The list of specific causes is long: an improperly repaired meniscal tear or the removal of a meniscus, a fracture, bowlegs or knock knees, any abnormal development of the hip, prolonged immobilization, overuse of a joint that is not entirely normal, chronic inflammation or infection, and most rheumatic diseases, which means that osteoarthritis may actually be caused by rheumatoid arthritis. Certain diseases may also predispose one to OA, including diabetes and hypothyroidism.

One of the most important lessons we've learned in recent years regarding OA is that it is not a natural process of aging, nor is it necessarily a consequence of wear and tear. Consider, for example, that a whale, which spends its life supported in water in a total non-weight-bearing state, may have extensive OA while landlocked humans show no correlation between lifelong, weight-bearing physical activity and joint deterioration—even jogging does not lead to OA (see Chapter 19).

Rheumatoid Arthritis (RA)

Rheumatoid arthritis is a puzzle to researchers. RA is an inflammatory disease that is characterized by attacks on healthy tissue. The disease begins when the synovium (the thin membranes lining the body's joints) become inflamed. This inflammation may spread and destroy cartilage or weaken ligaments. RA is the most destructive form of arthritis. Whereas most forms of arthritis affect only a few joints, RA can cause damage throughout the body. It may even invade other body tissue, such as the heart or lungs. RA tends to be symmetrical, that is, joints on both sides of the body will often be involved. (However, one knee may be more severely diseased than the other.)

The effects of RA differ from person to person, but they often begin as mild symptoms that come and go before becoming chronic. Early in the disease process people feel tired, sore, achy, and stiff. The joints stiffen, then swell, and later become tender, making full motion difficult and painful. The knees, hands, and feet are the most commonly involved joints. Symptoms are generally most noticeable after long periods of inactivity, such as in the morning.

The most crippling effects of RA are seen in about one of every six RA patients. These people will experience severe aches, pains, and badly damaged joints. If the hands are severely affected, the fingers may become crooked and deformed so that movement is difficult.

Rheumatoid arthritis (RA), often occurs in younger individuals and even children. Unlike OA, which tends to be seen more often in men, women have the leading edge for rheumatoid arthritis. Of the six million Americans suffering from RA, three out of four are women between the ages of twenty and fifty.

Gout

Gout is the result of inflammation of the joints produced by an excess of uric acid. Usually, uric acid circulates in the blood as a by-product of normal metabolism and gets whisked away through the kidneys. Gout patients, however, either produce too much uric acid or the kidneys can't process and remove it properly. Either way, the end result is a uric acid buildup in the form of needle-sharp crystals of monosodium urate in the joints.

The damaging mechanism of gout is a combination of erosion and inflammation. Those crystals are deposited in the cartilage and synovium, which we just defined as the starting spot of RA. This causes acute and chronic inflammation and, over time, an erosion of the cartilage and the underlying bone.

Gout is far more common than most people think. Nearly two million people in the United States suffer from it, 95 percent of whom are men. Acute gouty arthritis usually appears without warning, often at night, and may follow overindulgence in food or alcohol, fatigue, and emotional distress. The pain is not easily ignored and is often described as throbbing, crushing, or excruciating. It may be so severe that even the pressure of a thin bed sheet can not be tolerated. The inflammation often resembles an acute infection: there is swelling, warmth, redness, and extreme tenderness. Although the classic location for gout is generally considered to be the big toe, it also commonly affects the knee, instep, ankle, wrist, and elbow.

The first attack of gout may last only a few days, but if left untreated, subsequent attacks may last for weeks. While gout is generally asymmetrical, that is, limited to one foot and not the other or one knee and not the other, the onset is rapid compared to osteoarthritis. It's even easier to distinguish gout from rheumatoid arthritis since RA is more likely to be symmetrical, more gradual in onset, and more likely to last longer for each acute attack.

Systemic Lupus Erythematosus (Lupus)

We'll briefly mention one other common rheumatoid disorder that may affect the knees, systemic lupus erythematosus. Called SLE or lupus for short, this is another rheumatic disease that affects many more women than men. It is mild for many patients but it can lead to serious problems, including damage to the skin, joints, and internal organs.

There is no known cure for lupus, but the treatment program can help reduce pain and inflammation and prevent serious joint damage from occurring. The treatment includes medication, heat or cold treatments, exercises, rest, joint protection, and, because of a sensitivity to sunlight, which often accompanies this disease, avoiding sun exposure.

DIAGNOSING ARTHRITIS

It's important to distinguish everyday aches and pains from the onset of arthritis because early detection can prevent permanent damage. Warning signs include:

—persistent pain and stiffness upon awakening or at the end of the day
—pain, tenderness, or swelling in one or more joints
—inability to move a joint normally
—recurrent or persistent pain and stiffness in joints
—symptoms such as these that last for more than six weeks.

Making an accurate arthritis diagnosis, however, is not always easy. Prompt medical attention may prevent irreversible damage, but it may take a couple of weeks to several months to achieve a detailed diagnosis. If your personal physician is unable to arrive at an accurate diagnosis, you should be referred to a rheumatologist (a physician who specializes in the diagnosis and treatment of all forms of arthritis).

In addition to physical examinations, physicians use tests to assist in the diagnosis of arthritis, including X rays, blood tests, joint fluid analysis, and examination of small samples of muscle or joint tissue. X rays can show revealing changes in the joints and blood tests can indicate whether a complex protein called rheumatoid factor or elevated levels of uric acid are circulating in your bloodstream. Joint aspiration and tissue biopsies are not the most comfortable tests you'll ever find in a doctor's office, but they can be critically important in establishing the definitive diagnosis.

There may soon be additional means of diagnosing arthritis. We've discussed the growing role of magnetic resonance imaging (MRI) in the diagnosis of knee problems. Eventually MRI may replace arthrography and arthroscopy, which are also occasionally used in the diagnosis of OA and RA. MRI may offer a great advantage in the diagnosis of arthritis patients who report pain but do not yet have clinically recognizable signs of disease. This is a particularly frustrating phenomenon early in the course of the disease. Just when medical intervention may be most successful, arthritis is most difficult to diagnose.

Another new technology may soon let doctors hear your body talk. By tuning in to the vibrations a joint makes when it moves, by listening for that nearly inaudible crackle like crumpled plastic that reveals early arthritis, doctors may be able to detect arthritis in a noninvasive manner even before some of the current invasive approaches can be successfully utilized. Many of us are unnerved by the snap, crackle, pop of our joints, but that's not really related to arthritic changes. To the human ear the sounds of arthritis really are the sounds of silence. It takes an inexpensive ($200) device called a rectifying-demodulating phonopneumograph (mercifully shortened to RDP) to listen in on your joint complaints. The microphone picks up inaudible sounds and produces a graph that displays a normal knee with both sharp peaks and smooth curves of sound or an arthritic knee, which graphs out with only sharp multipointed peaks.

While we still have no known cure for the major rheumatic diseases, the significance of what we have learned is substantial. If arthritis is not inevitable or a necessary consequence of activity, then there must be ways to interrupt the process, manage the disease, and possibly reverse it. We'll take up the rest of this story later in our section on relief and rehabilitation.

PART TWO

What to Do About It:
Relief and Rehabilitation

8

Questions to Ask Your Doctor

The most common complication in medicine is poor doctor/patient communication. It's especially problematic for knee patients because few have had much exposure at all to orthopedics. What do you ask? What do you say? And more fundamental yet: Who should you go to see?

ARE YOU THE RIGHT DOCTOR FOR ME? FIND OUT!

When you decide to see a doctor you may first visit your family practitioner. This approach has some advantages: It's probably cost-effective, you have good access, the doctor knows your medical history, and probably has some important insights into you as a person as well as a patient. However, if your doctor feels the need to inject you with cortisone, immobilize you in a cast or brace, or recommends physical therapy, you may wish to consult an orthopedist. The first two approaches may simply cover up the symptoms, while the last one could actually compound the problem in the absence of a complete and clear diagnosis. In any event, if after a few days you show no distinct signs of improvement, it's definitely time to get a second opinion.

This is not so much a reflection on your own doctor's capabilities as it is an indication of the complexities surrounding this medical specialty. Simply put, the doctor who is best at treating life-threatening problems may *not* be the one to get your bum knee back to work. The examination of an acutely injured knee can be very difficult and misleading, even to an experienced clinician. So you need to find a doctor who has managed to keep up with the changes and whose knowledge is based on experience, not just a review of the literature.

If you suspect you're going to need a specialist, instead of asking your doctor for a generic referral, ask a specific question: "Who would you send a member of your family to if they had a knee problem?"

Take your doctor's advice and contact the person suggested. But at the same time tell your doctor that you would like to ask friends and associates for recommendations. Then ask if your doctor would be willing to review the list of suggestions and help you make a choice.

Ask your sources how they found their doctor. Are they satisfied with the treatment they received? What problems have they experienced? And, most important, ask, "How's your knee?" Have they recovered or simply decided to live with a serious knee deficiency? A lack of pain is one thing, a complete recovery and return to active participation is quite another. Find out what their particular knee problem happened to be, then look it up in these pages. Was it a truly serious injury that would explain their lack of performance, did they neglect their rehabilitation program, or did their doctor simply go on to other patients, leaving this one to hobble into the ranks of the seriously impaired?

A good health club, a well-designed and -managed aerobics class, friends or associates who are deeply involved in sports, a sports specialty store—any of these sources could provide you with referrals to competent sports medicine experts. But again, check the names with your family doctor. The runner's store may merely suggest a favorite doc who happens to do a great 10K run or the ski shop may give you the name of a physician who recently ran up a $500 tab on a major shopping spree.

Once you come up with a name or two, the best approach is a face-to-face meeting. You're entering into a relationship with another human being and a lot can be learned from the rapport that can come only from personal contact.

First, of course, you need to phone the doctor's office. Before you even make an appointment you might want to ask about office hours and insurance acceptability. You can also quickly ask if the physician is board-certified, the percentage of his or her practice that is knees, and if he or she is a member of any special societies, such as the American Orthopedic Sports Medicine Society or the North American Arthroscopy Association.

While you wait for your meeting you'll be surrounded by people who can give you inside information. Start a conversation by saying that you're new and would appreciate any information they might offer regarding this physician or this office, in the case of a group practice. Besides questions about the surgeon, find out if they've ever had problems getting an appointment. Ask if they've ever called the office after hours. Was there a prompt response? Most people will be flattered that you asked and the ensuing discussion will undoubtedly be more educational than the dog-eared magazines you could be reading. If you have a general reluctance to enter into conversations in doctors' offices, remember that this is the ideal setting: Bum knees are not considered a communicable disease.

Once inside the hallowed halls of orthopedia, don't hesitate to ask questions. Here's a starter list:

Where did you go to medical school?

Where did you do your orthopedic training and was it an accredited program? (The American Board of Orthopedic Surgery evaluates various residency programs to make sure that they fit their criteria of exposure to all aspects of orthopedics, including trauma, reconstructive surgery, pediatric surgery, hand surgery, etc., and in order to become qualified for a certification in orthopedic surgery, the surgeon must be a graduate of an approved program.)

Are you specially trained in sports medicine or have you gone through any fellowship programs?

Approximately how many knee surgeries do you do in a year?

If surgery is one of your options: What is your success rate with this particular surgery? (If the answer is 100 percent, you've probably got the wrong surgeon. There is no 100 percent in medicine—no guarantees, no warranties. If you can't trust a surgeon to answer a simple question honestly, do you really want to put your life in his or her hands?)

If the surgeon is in a group practice: Do your partners cover you in the event of an absence?

If it's a solo practice: Who's on call when you're unavailable? Again, you want to know the background of these people if they're likely ever to care for you.

You will most likely be charged for an office consultation. However, if you use this approach to find a good doctor or to avoid one you're not gong to be happy with, this will be a good investment of both time and money.

ARE YOU DOING THE RIGHT THING?

If special diagnostic tests are recommended, once again you need to know the experience behind the procedure. The two centers that we use for magnetic resonance imaging have an accuracy of about 90 percent in diagnosing meniscal tears. A number of other centers we have evaluated have an accuracy rate of 70 percent. And I daresay there are new MRI facilities opening all the time that probably have even less success merely because they don't have the experience yet. Ask your surgeon. He should know the accuracy of the specialists he's sending you to for the tests.

Ask for the rationale behind any particular test that is recommended. Also, find out as much as you can about what the test entails. Various studies have shown that the more familiar a patient is with a test the less anxiety and discomfort they'll experience. Will it hurt? How long will it take? How will I feel afterward? Is it invasive? Do I have to drink something or is something injected into me? Who will do it?

One of the few questions patients consistently think to ask is "Will it hurt?" Regarding the question of pain, it's interesting to note that the doctor may not be the best one to ask. Researchers at the University of California, San Francisco, found that health professionals tend to seriously underestimate the physical and mental impact of tests on patients. After all, they may not fully appreciate what the patient is experiencing if they've never undergone the procedure themselves. On the other hand, the same study found that patients tend to overestimate the discomfort they would experience, preparing for the worst. It would be a good idea to read

Chapter 9 and learn about the tests you might have recommended to you.

WHAT ABOUT SURGERY?

Once the subject of surgery is brought up, ask: "What are the risks of this procedure?" You have to ask the question, although keep in mind that your doctor's answer may be of questionable value. In a survey reported in *The Western Journal of Medicine*, physicians and surgeons were asked to estimate the risks associated with ten common procedures. The results were almost evenly divided between those who were correct, those who underestimated the risks, those who overestimated the risks, and those who simply said they didn't know. Even worse, this distribution is typical of people who are guessing. (By the way, experience or board certification had little influence on the survey results.) If you ask a question regarding the risks of surgery and the response sounds more like a dismissal than an answer, ask for specifics. Only then will your surgeon look up the information and learn the answer.

If surgery is recommended, where will it be performed? If it's a hospital, what type of facility is it? Is there an intensive care unit, a coronary intensive care unit, pediatric intensive care unit? These would suggest an institution with a full range of capabilities. You hope you won't need it, but if you do, is the emergency room staffed by moonlighting physicians trying to make some extra money or is it a full-time emergency-room staff? Who will do the surgery? That may sound like a strange question to ask a surgeon, but if the orthopedist has a teaching center with residents and fellows, you really should know whether the orthopedist or a first- or second-year resident will be doing your surgery.

Often a surgeon is assisted during surgery. Who will be in the operating room with you? Will it be a nurse assistant, physician's assistant, another doctor? What is the assistant's experience? Will it be a family practitioner who is assisting for the supplemental fee or is it a really qualified assistant for this particular surgery? Will it be a nurse anesthetist or an anesthesiologist? Will you be able to discuss anesthesia before the operation?

Today you're as likely to have surgery performed in an outpatient center as you are within a hospital. To check the credentials of this facility, call and ask if they are Medicare-certified. This is a hallmark used by many insurance companies to determine their reimbursement, because Medicare certification is actually based on tougher standards than most state licensing boards. Also, ask if they have received accreditation from the Joint Commission of the AAAHC. The former, which is actually the Joint Commission of Accreditation for Hospitals, is the same body that provides accreditation for hospitals and now does the same for freestanding surgical centers. The Accreditation Association of Ambulatory Health Care (AAAHC) is a voluntary association that provides three-year, two-year, one-year, or no accreditation to surgical facilities. The three-year accreditation means that the center has fully met the AAAHC standards and passed inspection. A two- or one-year accreditation means that the facility may provide care but there are problems that the AAAHC will review later to determine whether the center then meets their strict standards.

What About Second Opinions?

Of course before there's any cutting done, you may wish to get a second opinion. Your first source should be the surgeon you're talking to: What are the alternatives? For example, your surgeon recommends diagnostic arthroscopy. You ask, "What do you expect to find?" "Probably a torn ligament." "What will my treatment be?" "We'll get you into rehabilitation and see how it goes." "What if I don't have the arthroscopy?" "Well, we'll put you into rehabilitation and see how it goes."

By asking a critical question—"How will the procedure change my treatment?"—you may decide to forgo the procedure at this time.

If you decide to seek an outside opinion, this is a fine way to confirm your medical situation and the surgeon's recommendations. The second opinion should be obtained from a board-certified orthopedic surgeon with the same expertise as your original orthopedic surgeon. This means that if your first doctor's specialty is knees, the second opinion shouldn't come from a back specialist. If your first surgeon is reluctant to help you seek a second opinion, I'd find another surgeon.

Of course second opinions can also be confusing. What should you do if the opinions disagree? The mere fact that there is a disagreement does not necessarily mean your surgeon was wrong. If there is a disagreement, ask the second surgeon for details regarding his conclusion. What course of treatment would he recommend? If the surgery is delayed, would it still be an option later? If you are uncomfortable with the differing opinions, ask if there is a recognized specialist who could be consulted regarding your specific case. Frankly, that's not often necessary. A second opinion is like getting a second bid on a car loan or another estimate of how much it will cost to remodel your house. The decision is not based on what you want to hear but on what you believe to be appropriate after considering both sides.

Finally, before you go into surgery you should ask questions regarding rehabilitation. Unlike having an appendix removed, which will require some medication and a few days to get back on your feet, orthopedic surgery requires the active participation of the patient in the recovery process. What will be required of you after the surgery? How much rehabilitation will be necessary and for how long a period of time? If you neglect your rehabilitation program, what are the complications that could result? Without appropriate rehabilitation, patients may actually be in worse shape after surgery than they were before.

9
What Are You Doing to Me?

It was not too long ago that knees, like backs, were a diagnostic mystery. For backs, there is a diagnosis called lumbar myalgia, which is a $250 word that means your back hurts. We had a similar diagnosis a few years ago in sports medicine: internal knee derangement, or I.D.K. The joke among specialists at the time was that those initials actually stood for "I Don't Know." Today, 95 percent of the time, we do know.

Keep that in mind when you limp into the examining room for the first time. You may feel a bit intimidated when you enter our strange and wonderful diagnostic world; you'll think it's strange, we think it's wonderful. You may even feel like decking the first person who touches your knee, but trust me. We're not sadistic demons out to introduce you to whole new plateaus of agony. Here's what we diagnosticians have to do to you—and why.

The most important diagnostic tool a good examiner has is a careful history of the problem as given by the patient. What doctors look for is the character (sharp, dull, aching, radiating) and location of pain in as much detail as possible. Is the pain related to activity? Does it occur only during activity or does it also occur at rest? Your doctor will often be as interested in past trauma as he or she is with current events. Sometimes what appears to have caused your problem merely accentuated a chronic condition. So if you think about these questions before you visit your doctor, you'll have a better idea of what information your doctor needs and a better idea of how to communicate your particular problem.

The physical examination will generally include observation of your gait. You'll walk a few steps, and in some cases that will halt the knee examination right there. Some back and hip problems can "refer" pain to the knee, so in these cases the real problem is not in the knee at all.

When we examine the extremities we usually have a standard for comparison. This can be very valuable. I've examined patients with several degrees of extra movement in their injured knee, and I'm ready with a diagnosis, only to find that their "normal" knee has the same movement. These individuals were just built a little differently.

After observing the appearance of the injured knee and comparing it with its uninjured partner, the physician manually checks for areas of tenderness. This can reveal a lot about the actual injury (or injuries). Also, if the site of pain changes with motion, this can distinguish one injury from another. For example, traveling tenderness during movement is more indicative of ligamentous injury as the ligament moves forward and backward with knee motion. A fixed location of tenderness, despite a change in knee position, is more typical of a meniscal injury.

There are several simple tests for knee stability. One of the simplest is to gently hyperextend the relaxed knee. A response of pain may indicate a meniscal tear. *McMurray's test* may also be used to check for meniscal damage: This is where the patient lies facing the ceiling and the knee is flexed. The physician keeps one hand on the knee while rotating the foot and slowly extending the knee, listening or feeling for a click as the femur passes over the meniscal tear.

There is also an *anterior drawer test.* If you wonder what cabinetry has to do with a knee examination, keep that drawer in mind for a moment. In most cabinets, if you pull the drawer forward, or anteriorly, there is a restraint that stops the drawer from coming all the way out. If the anterior cruciate ligament has been damaged, it will allow the knee to come forward more and more with the degree of damage. Likewise, if you shove a drawer back into a

McMurray's test

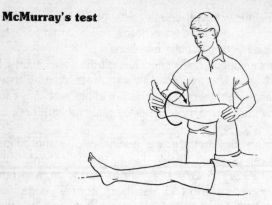

cabinet, there is a restraint stopping it from going all the way back and crashing into the wall. If the posterior cruciate ligament is damaged, the knee will go back posteriorly farther than normal.

So, again with the patient supine, the physician flexes the knee to about ninety degrees and anchors the foot, usually by sitting on it. The knee is gently pulled anteriorly (forward) and then posteriorly (backward). If there is significant displacement of the tibia on the femur, the test is positive and a torn cruciate ligament is suspected.

Anterior drawer test

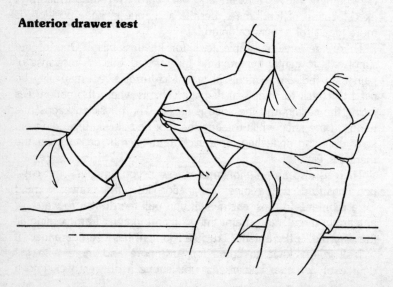

After years of experience with the drawer tests, a doctor in Philadelphia developed his own technique, which is now considered even more sensitive for determining cruciate ligament integrity. For the *Lachman test,* the examining physician holds the leg up and keeps the knee flexed at about twenty degrees while checking for anterior and posterior displacement.

Lachman test

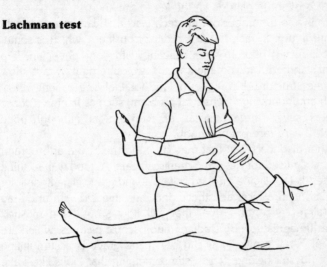

Simpler still is a little test to detect subtle areas of weakness. Most physicians will have you extend your leg and check your ability to lift against a slight pressure. I have learned a little trick from Dr. James Nicholas in New York City that is an even better indicator of muscle strength. I ask the patient to bend their knee; if they're seated, I'll have them lift one leg and resist as I push down on their thigh. Because the quadriceps are so strong, this test manages to change their leverage, make them relax, and allows me to detect even subtler signs of weakness. I'm not pressing on the knee, remember, so this is not very painful.

There is also finely calibrated technology that can detect such weakness. A *Cybex machine* is capable of detecting minute leg-strength discrepancies and, with the help of a computer printout, allows us to follow precisely the patient's progress. (This technology is discussed in further detail in the rehabilitation section.) A smaller, office version can also detect subtle differences. But for many patients a simple low-tech approach is all that is necessary. Occasionally, if there is no detectable weakness, I may question whether there really has been a knee injury. Muscle weakness associated with injury develops so fast that if there is not some definite muscular deficiency apparent, I might look more for a hip or back problem that is referring pain down the leg to the knee.

There is also a number of high-tech tests that can give us insight into your injury. In fact, the first order of business, which is sometimes conducted prior to even meeting with your physician, is a series of standard X rays of the knee. Yes, you're right, X rays show only bone structure, but we're looking for that one patient out of ten with an underlying mechanical problem, such as fractures, loose fragments, severe areas of wear, or even tumors, although bone cancer is a very rare phenomenon.

Another diagnostic test that may be performed is an arthrogram. It is primarily used for detecting meniscal tears. A good way to think of this test is to imagine mashed potatoes and gravy. The knee joint is numbed with a local anesthetic and then injected with an X-ray gravy (air or a contrast dye) that will flow around the mashed potatoes (knee tissue). By studying fluoroscopic pictures, which are a type of X-ray movie, you can see if the gravy is accumulating where it doesn't belong. If you see something that looks like Lake Michigan, well, that's normal. However, if you see something that looks like the Hudson River flowing out of Lake Michigan, you know you've got a problem. More than likely there has been a separation of the mashed potatoes (meniscal tissue) and it demonstrates a tear. The arthrogram is approximately 90 percent accurate on the inner side of the knee and slightly less accurate when viewing the outer side. Swelling is the only common side effect and complications are very rare. Because the contrast material has to be injected into a knee that is probably already painful and swollen, this is not a procedure most people would enjoy on a repeated basis.

Within the next few years the arthrogram will most likely be replaced by magnetic resonance imaging, which will probably be as important for the next century as the X ray has been for this one. The MRI imager looks like a giant empty spool of thread and it makes the body "broadcast" its condition to a team of radiologists and diagnosticians. The secret behind this internal radio show is a superconducting magnet 7,000 times stronger than the earth's magnetic field. The magnetic force causes protons in your body to turn left and right like little soldiers and emit a frequency signal that is picked up by an antenna and fed into a computer, which recreates images of the body. The technology provides precise images of soft body tissue and is becoming so sophisticated that we can almost see blood cells within blood vessels. It's as accurate as an arthrogram, if not more so, and offers the added advantage of imaging bony structures, ligaments, and tendons. And there's no pain involved, no side effects, and no X-ray exposure. The only thing you will be exposed to is a significant fee: $500 is average, but that's down from $1,500 just a couple of years ago.

Some doctors use computerized axial tomography, or CAT scans, to examine the position of bones and soft tissue. The CAT scan is a highly sophisticated form of X ray, 100 times as sensitive as a normal X ray, yet because the X-ray beam is extremely narrow, actual X-ray exposure may be less. This technology has been used primarily to evaluate the alignment of certain structures within the knee, muscle volume, and bone tumors. An injection of contrast material is also necessary for CAT scanning. An allergic reaction to the dye is the only possible side effect. If you have any known allergies, especially to iodine or fish (which is high in iodine), let your doctor know. Again, it looks like the MRI will replace the CAT scan.

Of course the best way to visualize some knee problems is by going in and taking a look. Once this little peek meant major surgery, a week in the hospital, and months of recovery. Today it may mean an outpatient procedure and immediate remobilization. Arthroscopy uses a fiber-optic telescope that allows the orthopedic surgeon to visually inspect the interior of the knee. Diagnostic arthroscopy has a high degree of accuracy and has spared many the trauma of exploratory surgery. It is an expensive procedure, however, costing anywhere from $1,200 to $2,000 for the surgeon's fee alone.

The arthroscope has a self-contained light source and can "railroad" cutting instruments into and out of the knee so that arthroscopic surgery can also be performed and leave the patient with nothing more than three puncture wounds about the size of a ballpoint pen refill. (For more details about arthroscopy see Chapter 12.)

There were 650,000 arthroscopic procedures done in the United States in 1985, according to figures from the National Center for Health Statistics. However, there were nearly 8 million office visits to orthopedic surgeons for knee problems, so obviously we can tell a lot about what's happening inside the knee from the outside.

Earlier we mentioned that fluid sometimes has to be removed from the knee by means of needle aspiration in order to check for some form of arthritis or infection or some other factor that could be causing swelling or effusion. Frankly, this is not a common clinical test. If you were to ask a rheumatologist who specializes in disorders such as arthritis, he'd probably do a sizable number of needle aspirations. And some nonorthopedic doctors may do aspirations almost as a reflex; they see something swollen, so they take down the swelling. But most orthopedists want to know, "Why is it swollen?" Swelling, or effusion, in a knee is like a cough. I could take a lot of time to study the cough, but it's not likely to tell me why you're coughing: Is it pneumonia, allergies, tuberculosis, or because you smoke too much? Swelling is secondary to something else. My job is determining what that something else is and for that I need to do a physical examination, take some X rays, look inside the knee, and get more information about what's going on in there.

There's another good reason for not doing a lot of needle aspirations. Although they are done under local anesthesia, they can still be painful. Unlike a tooth, which a dentist can easily numb, the knee contains several layers of skin, fat, muscle, and tendons. The lining to the joint may be very sensitive. So the whole area can't successfully be anesthetized.

Likewise, the injection of anti-inflammatories such as cortisone has changed considerably over the last five years. Once it was common to complain of knee pain and get a cortisone shot to deaden the pain. There are still times when a physician wants to be Dr. Feelgood; he or she wants to make the patient comfortable. But we have to be much more judicious about our use of such drugs today because of the large number of papers that have been published detailing the disadvantages of this approach. Cortisone changes the metabolism of the knee surface and it alters the body's inflammatory response. Over time this can cause progressive degeneration, and it exposes people to certain risks. Pain is a warning that says "Watch it!" And if that warning is not there, people may not be very careful.

There is still a limited place for cortisone. Sometimes I will use one or two injections to get patients over a difficult period in their recovery, if, for example, I've taken care of the mechanical problem but the joint is still inflamed. Some surgeons will inject cortisone immediately before surgery in an attempt to limit the inflammation response to the procedure. Others may look inside and find that the whole knee lining is inflamed, so they may use a cortisone injection to allow the patient to enter into a treatment program sooner and with more comfort. But again the risk here is that too much activity in the face of too little pain may cause a patient to hurt himself further.

One other cortisone candidate may be the older person whose knee is in bad shape yet, for whatever reason. He or she is not a candidate for total knee replacement at this time. Under these circumstances I may give one to two cortisone shots a year. A year? Yes, one shot of cortisone generally provides three to four months of relief, then there's a gradual return to pain. I underscore that this period of relief is what most patients experience. For some patients a cortisone shot will last forever; for other patients it lasts until they get to the parking lot.

All of this gives you an idea of what's going to happen when you have an examination for knee pain. If you have a chronic knee problem and much of the above information sounds new to you, you might want to check in with your doctor. I would guess there are a lot of people who initially developed problems several years ago and who have the general impression that "There's really nothing that can be done for my knee." We're fortunate to have experienced a phenomenal period of technological growth and educational advancement in treating knees in just the last few years.

Just a few years ago a diagnosis that suggested surgery might have led to a decision to live with the problem because surgery simply wasn't very desirable. Today the situation is much different, much improved. Thanks to arthroscopy, surgery is not as debilitating as it once was. We also know a lot more about proper rehabilitation, which means for some patients, their continuing problem is related to the fact that they were simply never rehabilitated properly.

And things are still changing fast. I ask some of my patients to check back with me in a year and I won't charge them for the office call. I'm a researcher and I want to follow up and document their recovery or lack thereof. But, too, I know that we can still learn a lot in just one year and what we have problems with now may be solved by an advancement that we haven't considered yet.

10

Pain Pills and Potions

No two people suffer pain alike. Some do it stoically, some do it sympathetically, and some do it loudly, but almost all of us do it with a pill. Pain relief medication is a $1.7 billion-dollar-a-year business, but that doesn't begin to suggest the size of the entire pain market. According to data circulated by the makers of analgesics, nearly one third of all Americans have persistent or recurrent chronic pain. Each year such pain costs an estimated $80 to $90 billion in doctors' fees, drugs, compensation, and litigation and is responsible for the loss of 700 million workdays.

Pain is perhaps the most personal of all experiences. Its impact is intimately intertwined with an individual's emotions, moods, upbringing, and general outlook on life. My trying to tell you about my pain is an approximation at best, an exercise in futility at worst. For this reason alone, discussing pain and its management is a complicated task. Throw in the fact that most of our information about pain comes to us from today's multibillion-dollar corporate pill peddlers and one begins to appreciate the benefits of arguing something a little more cut and dried—like politics or religion. As it relates to sports medicine in general and knee pain in particular, however, pain relief does become a slightly more manageable discussion topic. But only slightly.

The first problem is the psychological component. People who are athletically active—not just athletes, but also people who participate in recreational sports and activities—often believe that an admission of pain is tantamount to failure. Less extreme views, which consider pain an admission of imperfection or the price for play, are equally unhealthy. Pain is the body's alarm system. Shutting off the alarm, without finding out what triggered the alert in the first place, is both foolish and dangerous. By turning off the pain—which is your body's way of saying "Hey, there's something wrong down here!"—you can take a minor knee problem and turn it into an activity-stopping, life-altering injury.

Another, more complicated problem is determining what's causing the pain. In the case of the knee, we've discussed at length in this book the dozens of factors that play a role in the problems and symptoms associated with knee pain. The best rule of thumb for pill poppers is, if pain persists beyond three days of self-medication, get a medical examination.

Of course if you are self-medicating, you need something to medicate yourself with, and manufacturers have certainly stepped in to offer you relief: There are more than 100 different products vying to relieve your pain. Such variety! Such selection! Such a smoke screen! Your choices are basically three: aspirin, acetaminophen, and ibuprofen.

ASPIRIN

It has been called the "prince of panaceas" and "the miracle in your medicine cabinet." It's the little white pill you take for granted—and for almost everything else from colds to cramps, from hangovers to headaches, from rheumatoid arthritis to rheumatic fever. Americans consume more than 80 million aspirin tablets a day, 16,000 tons a year, or roughly 175 tablets per person per year. It's one of the earliest painkillers known to man. Two thousand years ago, Hippocrates, the "father of medicine," told women of ancient Greece to chew the bitter leaves of the willow tree to decrease the pains of labor. Today the active ingredient in those leaves, salicin, has been refined, and now acetylsalicylic acid, or aspirin, is the most popular drug in the world.

Although its chemical structure is simple, we haven't come close to fully understanding just how aspirin works. Prostaglandins are chemical messengers that are involved, one way or another, in virtually every biological function, but when produced in excess they can trigger pain, fever, inflammation, and more. Apparently, aspirin blocks the manufacture of prostaglandins. Whatever it does, aspirin has enjoyed almost a century of popularity because it works.

Aspirin is the active ingredient in Anacin, Excedrin, and Bayer. Buffered aspirin is also available and promoted as "faster" and "gentler" than plain aspirin. Actual clinical trials, however, have shown no difference in the speed at which plain or buffered aspirin works. As for the claim that buffering protects the stomach, aspirin can indeed attack the stomach lining and cause irritation, especially at the high dosages that are required for an anti-inflammatory effect. But here again researchers studying the claim have found no difference in damage. If a tablet has a special coating that prevents it from dissolving until it reaches the small intestine, then there is protection from stomach upset. Enteric coating, however, is not the same as buffering.

Most people have heard that alcohol and aspirin don't mix; their combined irritating effects may be especially hazardous to one's gastrointestinal tract. Less well known is the fact that aspirin and vitamin C may have a similar synergistic effect. Vitamin C is ascorbic acid and it is in and of itself a bit of an irritant to the stomach. When combined with aspirin, these two substances may be anything but healthy. If you're taking vitamin C, give the aspirin three hours to clear out of your stomach. And always take any analgesic with a full glass of water or other liquid in order to minimize any stomach upset.

Another side effect of aspirin is of special interest to anyone about to undergo a surgical procedure such as arthroscopy. Aspirin causes platelets, the disc-shaped clotting factors in blood, to become "slippery." These slippery platelets don't form clots, which can be beneficial as a protection against stroke but hazardous to surgical patients, who need their blood to clot in order to halt the bleeding caused by surgery. Thus *you should refrain from taking aspirin or other anti-inflammatory agents during the week prior to surgery.* If this presents a problem, it should be discussed with your physician.

Aspirin is so commonly used by athletes, I think some people get the idea that aspirin *is* sports medicine. A few years ago some researchers were actually suggesting that we increase our use of aspirin in sports. The theory was that aspirin might prevent cartilage damage by inhibiting certain destructive enzymes. Further study, however, has failed to confirm those initial findings. At the other extreme, some sports medicine specialists are now trying to get aspirin out of the locker room. Many athletes take aspirin to relieve the pain of injuries both big and small and they end up taking ten to twenty tablets a day. One football player who took up to fifteen tablets a day for more than a week ended up with small skin hemorrhages all over his body. This was a result of aspirin's ability to thin the blood. Does this mean we should get rid of aspirin in favor of some other pain medication? No. Anything—and especially any drug—taken to excess is bound to be harmful. This argues in favor of medical supervision, not against the use of aspirin.

ACETAMINOPHEN

The most popular aspirin substitute is acetaminophen (Tylenol, Anacin-3, Panadol, Datril), which does not cause as many gastrointestinal problems as aspirin but it also doesn't offer aspirin's anti-inflammatory effect. Still, it has taken 45 percent of the painkiller market, one percentage point behind aspirin, which had a fifty-five-year head start. That market share, however, is more a testament to advertising success than clinical success. Because of the massive amount of advertising being done, it's best to remember who's paying for these ad campaigns. According to *Consumer Reports* (February 1987), all acetaminophen is created equal. If your brand is more expensive, you're paying for a massive ad campaign, not for more effective pain relief.

Coming up with powerful descriptors such as "extra-strength" is also a marketing ploy and should not be confused with reality. Most extra-strength pain relievers are just larger doses of the regular-strength drugs. For instance, two extra-strength Tylenol tablets equal three regular-strength tablets. And they offer little, if any, additional pain relief compared to the regular dose. The smallest effective dose of any drug is the dose that should be taken.

Such marketing ploys only serve to sell a product and overdose the consumer.

One group of people should avoid acetaminophen—active alcoholics. A Veterans Administration study recently found that acetaminophen can cause serious liver damage in alcoholics, even with moderate doses of the drug. The study leads me to believe that long-term use could even be hazardous to the livers of nonalcoholic patients taking as few as six extra-strength acetominophen tablets a day.

IBUPROFEN

The new kid in town does reduce inflammation as well as provide pain and fever relief, and apparently accomplishes its task with a stomach-upset profile that is better than aspirin but not quite as good as acetaminophen. Ibuprofen (Advil, Nuprin, Medipren, Ibuprin) has quickly garnered 9 percent of the nonprescription pain-relief market, although it is considerably more expensive than aspirin.

Are you getting anything more for your money? Maybe. Studies suggest that you may be getting some pain-relief advantages with ibuprofen. Research suggests that one 200-milligram tablet may bring slightly more pain relief than 650 milligrams (two regular-strength tablets) of aspirin or acetaminophen. Although ibuprofen manufacturers suggest two tablets should be taken if one doesn't work, there's no benefit to taking *more* than two tablets for normal aches and pains. Studies suggest that dosages above 400 milligrams don't increase the level or duration of pain relief except for arthritis, where up to 800 milligrams are used at a time.

For sports medicine use, ibuprofen may hold some slight edge over the competition. Studies suggest it may be better for treating soft-tissue injuries such as sprains and strains. However, as one specialist put it in an overview of these and other non-steroidal anti-flammatory drugs (*Sports Medicine,* 1986, 3:242–46), much of the pertinent world literature on the value and usefulness of these agents in the treatment of sports injuries is "conflictual, vague, and uninstructive."

It's still too early to tell, but one of the original concerns about ibuprofen was its deleterious effects on the kidneys. Large doses or continued use over time can reduce blood flow to the kidneys, creating a serious situation for people who already suffer kidney impairment. Those who should take ibuprofen only under a doctor's supervision include individuals on diuretics or patients with kidney disease, heart disease, severe hypertension, or cirrhosis of the liver. Elderly people, with or without these problems, could also face a risk since kidney function declines with age. Anyone who notices fluid buildup (edema), back pain, increased urination, or a change of color to their urine must contact a doctor immediately. These symptoms could be a sign of kidney damage.

CREAMS AND LOTIONS

How do they get heat in an ointment? Generally by making wintergreen a primary ingredient. This aromatic plant is a mild irritant and it causes the sensation of warmth. Some of the rubs also have Xylocaine in them, which is a superficial numbing medicine.

Analgesic creams are not in my trainer's bag—at least not anymore. In England I saw a soccer team once and all they had on the sidelines was a bucket of ice water and a sponge. When an athlete went down he would scream, "I need the sponge." At that the trainer would race across the field and slap the "magic" sponge on the player's sore spot. That sponge and water were as effective as everything I had in my trainer's bag! I could hand out Band-Aids and splints and analgesics, I could immobilize a shoulder or brace a knee, and I watched that soccer team in England and I brought back a sponge. I wanted to remind myself to check my motives at all times. Am I working to help the athlete or to impress the coaches? Or am I acting just to look good?

If creams or ointments make you feel better, then use them. Sometimes I suspect it's less the actual lotion than it is the act of rubbing the sore spot that really helps, especially if someone else applies it for you. Massage makes anyone feel more comfortable and relaxed, and it may even improve flexibility and help the body metabolize some of the waste products of the athletic event.

Which of these is best for you? Only you can tell, and in fact, even between two medications that are absolutely the same you may find that one works for you while the other doesn't. Why? Some people might say it's your imagination, but it's more complicated than that. Research on the placebo effect, which is how the body responds to chemically inert substances such as sugar pills, suggests that up to one third the benefit of certain medications could be attributable to a familiar size, shape, color, or name on a tablet. This is not imaginary, nor should it be denigrated. Such effects can encourage the body's own pain-relieving efforts, and anything that can boost the potency of analgesic medication is a real boon to people in pain.

Don't, however, bombard your body with a little of everything in hopes of overwhelming the pain. What you really may be doing is overwhelming your body and doing significant damage. Don't even mix aspirin with one of the aspirin alternatives. There is a growing fear that combining more than one analgesic may increase the risk of kidney damage, for example. A number of countries have banned multi-ingredient painkillers. The United States, however, is not one of them. Read the package before you buy a painkiller and check that you're not getting a mixed bag of medication.

Perhaps the biggest problem associated with all this self-medicating is a major new risk of ulcers. Over-the-counter analgesics, such as aspirin, are a fraction of the total market for non-steroidal anti-inflammatory drugs, or NSAIDS. Over 270 million prescriptions for NSAIDS are written each year. But whether prescription or over-the-counter, NSAIDS may be causing ulcers in an estimated 20 percent of the 40 million Americans who regularly use these drugs.

These ulcers associated with NSAIDS are often symptomless, providing no warning to the patient or physician.

Again, we've been so bombarded with advertising touting these products that we have become almost anesthetized to the fact that these are all powerful drugs. And in sports medicine we have already mentioned the risks involved with burying pain and steamrolling ahead with activity. Use of these drugs is certainly no substitute for the more permanent forms of rehabilitation we'll be discussing.

There is, of course, a time and place for pain relief in sports medicine. Sometimes you overdo it and need some relief from your complaining muscles; at other times, medication can ease recovery. And if you're in rehabilitation, pain relievers may reduce your discomfort and increase your chances of completing your therapy program. If you find a drug that works for you, fine, but if you find that you're relying more and more on medication, it's time to see a doctor before you suffer a mid-sports crisis.

11

Surgery?
The Pros and Cons

Sports medicine is capable of some pretty spectacular successes; unfortunately, there is no orthopedic condition that can not be made worse by surgery. This is not meant to scare you away from surgery. It is meant to underscore the seriousness of any surgery and remind you that, gee-whiz press reports aside, even arthroscopy—a type of surgery, remember—needs to be considered carefully, like any other surgical procedure. This means you need to understand your options and the risks that are involved. You need open communication with your surgeon and an honest assessment of whether you're going to be ready, willing, and able to proceed with the rehabilitation that is recommended. The most skillful execution of any type of knee surgery will not bring satisfactory long-term results unless it is followed by a good rehabilitation program.

Although arthroscopic surgery has saved hundreds of thousands of people from lifelong limps, there are some fears that it's being performed too frequently. We'll be discussing arthroscopy at length in the following chapter.

The sheer economics of surgery in general underscores the potential for overutilization. For an office call a doctor may get up to $100. If a decision is made to look inside the knee and check for damage, diagnostic arthroscopy can easily cost $750. Then if further surgery is required, that starts at about $1000 and goes up.

Fortunately, many insurance companies now pay for second opinions. So when you're told that surgery is the answer, no surgeon should balk if you decide it's time to ask someone else the question. Of course we've already mentioned that you could ask your own surgeon for a second opinion. Find out about alternatives. Your physician should first ask about your level of athletic participation and then take into account your age, life-style, and interest to return to specific activities. Once all of this has been determined you will generally face two options: an optimal result and an acceptable result. For the optimal result, surgery may indeed be necessary, along with a solid rehabilitation program. On the other hand, if your athletic goals are modest, then surgery may not be necessary. An acceptable result should mean no pain, full range of motion, and an ability to do light activity, such as bicycling, swimming, or doubles tennis.

You may also find that even if you decide against immediate surgery, it could still be an option at a later date. Remember, innovations in knee surgery outrun the textbooks printed to describe them. To be sure, ask your surgeon if postponing the procedure will make it more difficult or less likely to succeed at a later date.

A perfect example of this approach is a torn cruciate ligament. We once thought that an unrepaired torn anterior cruciate ligament would preclude future athlete participation and lead to progressive instability, progressive tears of the menisci, progressive disability, and progressive deterioration of the knee joint.

The fact is, knees can have an absent anterior cruciate ligament without any functional disability and very little instability. Also, research indicates that the absence of an anterior cruciate ligament does not preclude athletic participation, does not cause subsequent tears of the menisci, does not lead to progressive instability, and does not produce progressive joint deterioration.

Without surgery a patient with a torn ACL has an unstable but usable knee, assuming that he or she does not engage in strenuous athletics. The best example I can think of is me. I mentioned earlier in this book that I have a torn anterior cruciate ligament. I tore it when I was in high school. Today I ski and play racquetball. However, I have made certain adjustments in my style. I tend to lead with my best leg, for example. I've had four episodes of instability in twenty-five years, during which episodes I was playing football, skiing, or playing tennis. Each time the knee would shift out upon extension, roll back, and then swell up. Imagine a sliding door that goes off the track momentarily and then bounces back. Such episodes do not mean reconstruction to me. Four episodes in a year would, especially if they were brought on by activities of daily living.

You can compensate a little for damaged cruciates by building up the strength of your knee muscles. Overall, one third of all patients suffering an acute ACL injury will do well with rehabilitation plus proper bracing during athletic activity. Another one third will be borderline, and the final one third will have significant problems that will definitely require surgery. These figures could probably be improved if patients would only cooperate. The same study suggests that only 40 percent of these patients use their braces when they are supposed to and only 35 percent follow their rehabilitation programs.

So it seems reasonable that if disability persists despite adequate conservative treatment and muscle conditioning, then some surgical procedure directed at repairing or reconstructing the anterior cruciate ligament should probably be considered. (Reconstruction involves the use of either a natural or artificial ligamentous replacement.)

In short, there's no such thing as always and never in medicine. We must individualize. You might be a textbook candidate for surgery, but if we are convinced that you'll never maintain the follow-up conditioning program, then we have an obligation to seriously consider not putting you through an operation. On the other hand, if you're an active sports participant, we may decide to go in and repair even a relatively minor ligamentous tear.

Whether you decide to go with surgery or first try an alternative treatment, for the most part the success or failure you will face will be in your own hands. That's because with or without surgery the key to recovery is rehabilitation, and no matter how technologically superior we become, the significance of rehabilitation is not likely to diminish anytime soon.

12

Arthroscopy
Cut and Run

Picture a building. There are no doors, no windows, no entryway whatsoever. You don't know what's inside, but you have to find out quickly, someone's life could depend on your actions—or you could be wrong and there really is no emergency. You might decide to bide your time, hoping for news from inside, but eventually if you had to find out what was going on inside you'd have only one choice: crash through a wall.

For years that was the less than subtle approach surgeons had to take to find out what was happening inside a knee. A life was never at stake, but a person's life-style certainly was. Unfortunately, the pain, swelling, and disability that followed exploratory surgery created considerable reluctance to open up a patient. A wait-and-see approach was adopted. If the patient got better, fine, they avoided a major surgical procedure. But if there was no improvement, and in fact many got plenty worse, the surgeon would have no choice but to open the leg and take a look around. This certainly was one way to find out what was going on in those closed quarters called the knee. However, as this diagnostic procedure often required a recovery time longer than that required for the injury itself, the situation was ripe for a technological leap.

In the 1970s a Japanese surgeon perfected the arthroscope. The term comes from the Greek words *arthros* (joint) and *scopos* (to look) and literally means "to look within a joint." Finally, thanks to fiber-optic illumination and sold-state electronics we no longer have to crash through the wall just to see what is going on inside. Instead of cutting open the leg and slicing through muscle and other healthy tissue, we can now cut two small holes in the knee and peek inside with a telescopelike device.

The first hole, or portal, is for a cannula, or tube, which is slipped into the knee; sterile fluid is pumped through it to expand the space in the joint. Then the arthroscope is inserted from a second portal. This steel cylinder is the approximate thickness of a soda straw and from its tip gleams a brilliant, cool light. Attached to the arthroscope is a video camera. An eyepiece allows direct visual access or a TV monitor provides a magnified view.

At first the scope was only used diagnostically. If any work needed to be done, the surgeons went ahead and cut open part of the knee, but at least unnecessary damage was kept to a minimum. Then miniaturized surgical tools were developed, and through a third portal tiny clamps, forceps, scalpels, drills, and clippers could all be used in the knee.

Comparing arthroscopy with open surgery (arthrotomy) gives you an idea of just how far we've come: It's the difference between carpentry and watchmaking. With arthrotomy the patient faced a week of hospitalization, eight to twelve weeks of strenuous and painful rehabilitation, and got a zipperlike scar for a souvenir. Contrast that with arthroscopy, where patients are often seen on an outpatient basis, they're on their feet—on crutches—the very same day, and three little bandages cover the incisions, which are usually only a quarter of an inch across. Minimal pain and immobilization permit early and aggressive physical therapy.

Needless to say, all of this brings along an air of the miraculous. The lay public considers arthroscopy "Band-Aid surgery," and only a wimp or a four-year-old is afraid of a Band-Aid, so many people are absolutely fearless when it comes to arthroscopy. In fact, I'm actually left in the bizarre position of having to talk some patients *out* of arthroscopic surgery. They tell me they have to have surgery because a friend of a friend had the exact same problem and is now running the Boston Marathon—backward.

Back in 1985, while reflecting on the tenth anniversary of

arthroscopic surgery in the United States, Dr. Robert Metcalf put arthroscopy into perspective. During his presidential address before the annual meeting of the Arthroscopy Association of North America, he noted, "Arthroscopy is not an end in itself. Arthroscopy is a technique. It is a technology. It is a method of accomplishing end results that are less invasive, less destructive of normal tissues, more accurate, but more difficult than any procedure we have had for joint surgery."

It is important to remember that arthroscopy is not the surgical equivalent of "near beer"—it is real surgery with the same potential risks and complications inherent to any surgical procedure. The estimated complication rate for arthroscopic surgery ranges between 4 and 15 percent, depending on which study you read. A seven-year review of our own group's patients showed a rate of about 8 percent. Most of the complications are minor. The most common post-operative problem is hemarthrosis, which means joint pain and swelling caused by bleeding into the joint. This is often caused by the use of aspirin prior to or immediately after surgery, which prolongs bleeding in almost all cases. Hemarthrosis can result in increased scar formation, decreased range of motion, and synovitis, which all contribute to recurrent patellar disease. The signs of hemarthrosis include increasing pain and swelling, difficulty in straight leg raising, and at times a low-grade fever.

Postoperative effusion may also occur, and when it does it's often persistent. Quadriceps exercises begun prior to surgery and continued afterward have helped prevent effusion. Sometimes anti-inflammatory drugs are useful; occasionally a painful effusion needs to be drained.

Another complication stems from equipment failure, or more specifically (get ready to grimace) an instrument breaks off inside the knee. This is a pretty rare complication, but because the instruments are fragile and the knee is very tight, it's a real risk.

The biggest problem during surgery can be a pretty significant one: damage to cartilage. Once damaged, cartilage doesn't repair itself well and a bone can develop osteoarthritis.

What's the problem? A surgeon must learn to manipulate small, easily broken instruments inside a very tight joint while watching a magnified two-dimensional picture on a television screen. It's video-game medicine, Pac Man played for keeps. We're not talking carpentry here; if you make a bad cut, you can't just get another piece of wood. And if a surgeon lacks skills or patience, healthy cartilage or tissue can easily be scarred by a fumbled knife or a wrong move with a power cutter. If that doesn't cause you to blanch, think about the new technologies that are still experimental but likely to become standard equipment someday: lasers and high-speed motors. With these a surgeon loses the tactile feedback that tells him where the softened, damaged cartilage ends and the firmer, healthier cartilage begins. Without ever knowing it, a surgeon can cut a little too deep and single-handedly create an osteo-arthritic condition.

Even when arthroscopy is used diagnostically, it is still a surgical procedure. It is done in a standard operating room under sterile conditions, and usually with general or spinal anesthesia, although a local anesthesia is sometimes appropriate. It's accuracy as a diagnostic tool approaches 98 percent in skilled hands. Compare that to the clinical diagnostic accuracy of orthopedic surgeons, which ranges from 70 to 76 percent on average. For a technique developed outside the usual academic research settings, it's kind of stunning to realize that in ten years arthroscopy has worked its way into the hands of 7,000 to 9,000 orthopedic surgeons in North America and now accounts for 90 percent of all knee surgery in the United States.

Arthroscopy is most useful in evaluating and treating several specific knee problems. Once, for example, a torn meniscus was treated the same way we used to treat problems with the appendix: When in doubt, take it out. Now arthroscopy allows us to go in and take out only part of the meniscus. We run clippers, punchers, and shavers into the knee and the on-screen image has been described as "barracudas and snapping turtle heads biting away at a half flounder under a big white rock." That's certainly more descriptive than what surgeons call it: debridement.

Arthroscopy is also useful in diagnosing and managing certain ligamentous injuries. Bleeding inside the joint implies a cruciate ligament tear, and with a little skirting around various knee structures, it's easy to visibly inspect a torn cruciate ligament.

Remember, there are two types of ligaments—those on the sides of the knee joint (collateral ligaments) and those inside the joint (cruciate ligaments). Collateral ligaments can't be repaired arthroscopically; they require an incision into the knee. Back to our house analogy, we can't work on the collateral ligaments arthroscopically because they aren't just in the building (the knee) they are girders in the wall. The cruciate ligaments are increasingly being repaired by arthroscopy, but this is still regarded as experimental surgery and sometimes we have to open up at least a part of the knee. However, whether it's done arthroscopically or through an open incision, ligament surgery means a longer period of recuperation than does a cartilage removal.

So when a ligament needs to be repaired, the standard approach is actually a combination of arthroscopy and open surgery. This has caused a few patients to gulp. After all, this is one aspect of arthroscopy that hasn't gotten a lot of attention—it can't do everything!

It can help, however, when another cartilage problem arises. The articular cartilage on the underside of a normal kneecap is smooth. Occasionally, such as with patients who suffer chondromalacia, there may be a rough, eroded surface on both the patella and its neighboring femur. With the arthroscope we can go in and "shave" off the loose fibers and decrease some of the breakdown products that cause inflammation. This is a fairly new procedure, however, and operative results are too inconsistent to recommend this as an early approach. The best bet is a more conservative means of medical management. (See Chapter 5.)

Or cartilage can be worn and roughened by osteoarthritis. Fragments can even break off and go haphazardly around the inside of the knee, and these "loose bodies" can send your trick knee into all kinds of show-stopping acts. Arthroscopy can smooth roughened surfaces with power instruments and then suction out the debris. The underlying bone may also be abraded with a burr to stimulate cartilage growth.

Once the problem is outside the knee cavity, we're pretty much beyond arthroscopic capabilities. That means that problems such as patellar tendinitis or fractures of the patella would need an open surgical approach. Arthroscopy is also not capable of repairing an advanced arthritic knee, although this has more to do with the nature of the disease than any inherent deficiency in the technology.

Altogether, I'd say about 80 percent of my surgical procedures utilize standard arthroscopy, 15 percent are variations on the theme, meaning a mixture of closed and open procedures, and 5 percent are predominantly open surgery.

Although the incisions are small, people need to be reminded that they have had an operative procedure within the joint. Experience has shown that internal healing takes several weeks and, in fact, complete healing may take many months. In the case of major ligamentous damage, healing may take a year or more. If an arthritic condition co-exists with any knee problem, convalescence may be further lengthened.

You might find this quite difficult to accept. After all, you've probably heard about marathon runner Joan Benoit and gymnast Mary Lou Retton, who underwent arthroscopy shortly before qualifying for the Olympics. But rushing back to action too soon after surgery can cause reinjury. It's still surgery and it takes time, patience, and a lot of work to fully recover.

Finally, even basic procedures have up to a 10 percent failure rate. Failure is generally due to bad tissues, bad injury, bad healing, bad timing, or just bad luck. I've gone in expecting to find a real mess and I look around and it's not so bad. I have also gone in expecting a fairly cut-and-dried procedure only to find one complicating factor after another. Sometimes it just doesn't work.

That doesn't mean you can't try again. Sometimes we develop another plan of attack or consider a new technique. Maybe when you were first injured the new approach was still too experimental, but a year or two later it might be more refined. After all, arthroscopy is one of the fastest evolving medical specialties. New developments are emerging with great speed.

13

When All Else Fails:
Total Knee Replacement

Total knee replacement is a reality, but don't dream of bionic abilities matched only by Hollywood special effects. Such complete reconstruction is a radical solution to a dire medical situation. While the future looks promising, the current state of the art is far from ideal. The idea of replacing bad joints has gotten such breathless press that some people dismiss the damage they are doing to their knees, hoping for a bionic replacement. The news, however, is not quite so cheery. If your attitude regarding your knees is largely one of indifference, and if you expect a total joint replacement to mend the damage you are doing, you have seriously misplaced your faith.

The complexities of the knee make it one of the most difficult joints in the body to recreate, so we must underscore the seriousness of this particular solution to this major medical problem. The knee cannot, at this time, be duplicated.

Total knee arthroplasty (TKA), as it's called, is a means of repairing a knee that is seriously diseased and, despite every conservative therapy, has degenerated to where there is substantial disability and chronic pain. Usually the damage has been caused by rheumatoid arthritis or osteoarthritis.

About 100,000 total knee replacements are performed each year in the United States. Physicians prefer to limit this surgery to individuals sixty years of age or older and with good reason. Artificial joints may loosen over time or become infected and require replacement. Unfortunately, this is not a simple operation. It is a salvage operation that demands months of physical therapy to produce a successful replacement, which is still considerably disabling. Recipients must lead a very limited life-style. They can't jog, jump, climb, or squat. They can't play tennis, carry heavy loads, or work on uneven ground. Basically no pounding or heavy stresses are allowed at all.

We don't have a long history yet with this procedure, only about twenty years of solid experience. Of those that have been performed on forty- to fifty-year-olds, 85 percent have needed to be reoperated on within a decade (*The Physician and Sportsmedicine*, 14:6, 171–81, 1986). Subsequent operations have less bone to work with and what remains is of such poor quality that the likelihood of failure is even greater the second time around.

In general, the older you are, the better chance you'll have for a long-lasting replacement knee. Records show that older knee recipients have only a 3 percent chance of requiring further surgery. Why? If you're older, you're not likely to be as active, and thus there will be less stress on the knee. This is also why surgeons will generally try to delay the inevitable TKA with a number of other procedures. If the damage was created by rheumatoid arthritis, a synovectomy, or the total removal of the synovium, may buy the patient several years. (See Chapter 16.) A high tibial osteotomy, which is the knee realignment we've talked about before (See Chapter 5), may delay joint replacement by a decade or more, or it may preclude the need for the more extensive procedure.

If this sounds a bit frightening, it's meant to. I've seen too many knees, torn to shreds by sports, that could be mistaken for spaghetti. These young athletes, yesterday's gridiron heroes, now can look forward to hobbling around on pain-racked knees for thirty years or more, waiting to grow old enough to get an artificial knee.

While there are some 200 variations of total artificial knees available, all have been more successful in relieving pain for the severely afflicted person than simple medical management. If a surgeon is careful to select the right prosthesis and uses meticulous technique, 80 to 90 percent of patients may experience good to excellent pain relief. (Usually pain relief is not instantaneous. However, most patients obtain maximum pain relief within six weeks. Some patients, especially those with rheumatoid arthritis (RA), may still experience slight "barometric pain," which means their knees will still tell the weather.) Among the factors that influence the success rate of TKA are a patient's age, activity level, weight, and bone density.

Some surgeons report that patients with osteoarthritis (OA) often achieve better overall knee function than patients with rheumatoid arthritis, since RA patients are more likely to have additional joint involvement as well as muscle atrophy, weakness, and decreased ability to move around. However, because OA patients are likely to be more active than RA patients, some researchers suggest that loosening is more likely to be a problem with OA patients.

The surgery itself generally takes two to three hours. The prosthe-sis is comprised of three distinct parts. A metal cap, which is rounded to duplicate the bone itself, is attached to the end of the femur. The patella is replaced with a high-density polyethylene insert, which is then screwed or cemented to a base that is attached to the tibia.

Active physical therapy is usually begun within a few days of surgery; passive physical therapy, in the form of continuous passive motion (CPM), is often initiated within twenty-four hours of surgery. The benefits of CPM have only recently been recognized, and studies done at Brigham and Women's Hospital, Boston, suggest this improves the outcome of knee replacement surgery, shortens hospital stays, and improves flexibility. Within two weeks you're discharged, and by this time you should be able to walk using crutches or a walker.

If you're a candidate for a total knee replacement, you've probably had to avoid nearly all activity for years because of pain. So once you've had the surgery you may return to moderate walking, biking, cross-country skiing, swimming, horseback riding, ballroom dancing, bowling, rowing, gardening, or golfing—physician permitting. Light recreational cycling and swimming are encouraged because they are mostly non-weight-bearing activities. They are also valuable since heart disease may accompany the inactivity that caused the need for a total joint replacement. Aerobic activity, then, becomes a valuable adjunct for the younger artificial knee recipient.

New cementless prostheses, which actually allow bone to grow into the prosthesis, may significantly improve the prognosis for knee replacement. The key is the use of metal beads or fibers, which are placed on the implant, and bone actually grows in and around the spaces formed by these fibers and beads.

Besides promoting a better bond between the living bone and the inert artificial knee, the new procedure may also avoid the devastating infections that occasionally occur with the original replacement technology.

Like many complicated medical procedures, total knee replacement is not easy to do properly. If you are a candidate for a new knee, make sure that your surgeon has a lot of experience with this procedure. Since much of your life-style will depend on the outcome, you have a right to the best clinical experience.

I'm sorry to say bionic knees aren't going to have you leaping small buildings in a single bound or even outpacing a lethargic dog named Bullett, but for patients who have failed at a long list of more conservative therapies, total knee arthroplasty remains one glimmer of hope for a life-style that is racked by debilitating pain and chronic knee problems.

14

Rehabilitation:
The Achilles' Heel of the Knee

Whatever magic the surgeon's knife or the orthopedist's inventions may produce in a damaged knee, none of it is worth a plugged patella unless it's accompanied by an appropriate program to rebuild knee strength and endurance. Rehabilitation following surgery, for example, is now considered by many authorities to be of equal importance to the surgical procedure itself.

It hasn't always been this way. There was a time when sports medicine was aspirin, plaster of paris, and a strong recommendation away from strenuous activity.

Then science started to interfere with our practice of immobilizing every twisted knee. First evidence of disuse atrophy was found by the second postinjury day, along with a strength loss of up to 3 percent per day. Then researchers demonstrated that immobilization inhibits normal metabolic processes, which allows cartilage to maintain its toughness and resiliency. The end result is that parts of the knee quite literally starve. That's why when you take a cast off you find that your leg looks like it belongs on another body that's half the size of the one it's currently attached to.

Investigators soon theorized that early activity would increase blood flow, lessen vascular spasm, maintain a normal range of motion, and facilitate revascularization and the delivery of nutrients. A better understanding of physics, biomechanics, and other applied

sciences has allowed the development of an entirely new rehabilitative approach following major knee injury or surgery.

Unfortunately, people too often want a simple solution. They
want the pill that will make them better or the surgery that will solve
their problems, and physicians too often send patients off with a
poorly photocopied sheet of often unintelligible exercises or the
name of a local health club with the sage advice, "Don't overdo it."

Is it any wonder that the majority of the knee-injured are rehab
dropouts? They need information, support, and encouragement,
but instead they get referred, confused, and wholly frustrated.

Giving up is not, however, the answer. Insufficient or inappropriate rehabilitation is a leading cause of reinjury. Within a few months
of even a relatively minor injury, an unrehabilitated leg can lose half
of its strength, leaving that leg largely unprotected. Given that, what
constitutes a sufficient and appropriate rehab program?

There is no one blanket exercise prescription. You may have
special conditions that another person wouldn't have to be concerned with, such as old injuries or concurrent injuries. There are
some general guidelines, though.

SURGICAL REHABILITATION

Passive motion machines are now often used immediately after
surgery. These devices hold the leg and slowly keep it moving,
requiring no effort on the part of the patient. This protects against
early scar formation, which is one reason why casting creates a limb
that would not be out of place in the petrified forest. Anyone who
has ever had to have such scar tissue broken up during physical
therapy knows that there is something actually more painful than
their original knee injury.

After surgery specific rehabilitative exercises are recommended.
As soon as you can tense your quadriceps fifty times in succession
without pain, straight-leg raising is begun. As soon as you can flex
and extend your knee fifty times, from 90 to 180 degrees, then a
two-pound weight is added to your foot. One exception to this is if
you suffered serious ligament injuries; in that case exercise with
weights is limited or even avoided for the first six weeks and
strenuous exercises are avoided for the first three months of heal-

ing. Activities that have been shown to be safe include light swimming and exercise bicycling.

This approach has been so successful that many therapists are now backing up and providing a preoperative rehabilitation program. Physically, such a program better prepares the patient for surgery. Healing is facilitated and there is less need for rehabilitation after surgery. In fact, sometimes postsurgical rehab time is cut in half. Psychologically, a preoperative program of rehabilitation gives you confidence while limiting your fear and anxiety.

Altogether, this new approach to rehabilitation is changing the face of recovery. It has decreased the amount of hospitalization necessary, the severity of postoperative pain, and the utilization of medication. The early return to functional use usually means an earlier return to work. For example, the time off for a factory worker is cut nearly in half. Likewise, office workers are back at their desks in ten to twenty-one days after surgery, which is also one half of the time lost due to plaster casting.

As important as all of this is, there has been yet another advance in rehabilitation that is having a major impact on the treatment of sports medicine injuries. We can now precisely measure muscle function in terms of strength, power, and endurance. Once this was gauged by little more than educated guessing, but today an exact computerized printout of muscle function can be obtained using a Cybex (trademark) machine.

NON-SURGICAL REHABILITATION

Although we have emphasized surgical rehabilitation so far, few injuries are so minor that some form of rehabilitation is not necessary. Basically, any injury that keeps you from your favorite physical activities for as little as three or four days requires evaluation to make sure that function has not been impaired. Then, for every week of inactivity a conditioned body will require one month of rehabilitation to restore conditioning.

Emergency-room casts are now frequently thrown away as soon as a patient gets to his own physician. Instead, patients are given braces that strive for the optimal trade-off between immobility, which facilitates soft-tissue repair, and exercise, which facilitates revascularization and recovery. These braces allow flexibility but restrict injurious movement.

There are three phases to rehabilitation. The first—and shortest—is the early rehabilitation, or rest, phase, in which pain and inflammation are controlled with ice, aspirin, or an aspirin substitute and perhaps some of the rehabilitation technologies discussed later in this chapter. Even this "rest" phase includes mild exercise. For rehabilitation, rest is not the absence of activity but rather the absence of abusive activity. The intermediate phase is next and this includes more exercise to rehabilitate and rebuild strength and endurance. Finally, advanced rehabilitation includes conditioning for full functional performance in desired sports or activities, plus education on improving your exercise and activity form as well as how to train to avoid repeat injury.

REHABILITATING OLD INJURIES

For people like my co-author, who has walked around for at least three years with about a 40 to 50 percent muscle deficiency in his right leg, rehabilitation is appropriate even if there is absolutely no obvious muscular or joint insufficiency. This type of hidden weakness may be one of the biggest threats to knees today, especially considering the popularity of sports that require considerable knee action. Even worse is being weak in the knees and living a fairly sedentary life interspersed with periods of frantic activity— the feast-or-famine approach to exercise, which is so common among weekend athletes today and which makes knees extremely vulnerable.

However, if you aren't all that active, one vulnerable knee can still be your Achilles' heel. Even if my co-author weren't active, if he had injured his left knee instead of his right early in his running days, he more than likely would have hurt himself by now just getting out of the car. When a knee is that vulnerable, just twisting on it with your body's weight can cripple it. As it is, he has been lucky.

"What I don't understand," he said, shortly after discovering his one leg was at half strength, "is that this leg goes everywhere the other one goes. It's not like I unscrew my right leg every morning before I run." It's a rough one to understand, but daily living and even active living does not make sufficient demands on all the physiological systems supporting performance. Even running manages to exercise only a limited number of leg muscles.

Furthermore, once muscles have weakened, the body will adapt, and in that adaption it will prevent the muscles from ever recovering on their own. Indeed, this may have been very obvious in Rick's case. He admits that when he's driving he often finds his left leg is tensed. Although he dismissed this as a nervous habit, it's also possible to look at this as a coping mechanism. Such tensing is actually an isometric exercise. It's quite possible that his body is coping with the right leg's deficiency by making sure that the left side is strong enough to compensate. The problem comes if he ever has an accident: He could trip while running, step on an opponent's foot while playing basketball, or just take a misstep off of a curb and suddenly that weak knee will grab his attention in a most painful manner.

Or his knee might never bother him—but his back just might. When you favor a leg you're putting added stress elsewhere. This strain may not show up for years, but when it does we see a lot of patients complaining of back pain and wondering "What happened?"

"Does this mean I'm going to have to exercise this stupid leg for the rest of my life?" asks my co-author. (This from a man who doesn't think twice about possibly running for the rest of his life?) No, if you go through a three- to four-month program of exercise and progressive weight lifting, your right leg should become as strong as your other leg. If you were an athlete, however, whether high school, college, or pro, I might answer that question a little differently. In that case weight resistance exercise could be valuable for a year or more. Whether you're on the court or field every day or not doesn't matter; a daily program of weight-resistant exercises can be valuable following major injury. I've seen players carry on these exercises for two years or more and to definite advantage. Others have built up their musculature sufficiently to perform normal athletic chores and then stopped their exercise program only to have their rehabbed muscles waste away even while they play their sport daily. So for nonathletes a few months of rehabilitation following an old injury is probably sufficient and the muscles will recover and retain their strength. But for an athlete a longer maintenance program is probably most appropriate.

THE KEYS TO RECOVERY AND INJURY PREVENTION

Perhaps the single most important preventive and rehabilitative factor is body weight. Probably half of all knee patients could significantly ease their knee pain by achieving normal weight. Remember what we said about the extra weight that the knees must endure simply climbing stairs? For every ten pounds in excess weight, your knees have to absorb an extra forty pounds with each stair step.

Losing weight may also mean more oxygen is getting into the blood. If you hold your breath, your lungs don't appreciate that, and without enough oxygen they can start hurting fast. If you're overweight, the oxygen-carrying capacity of your blood may be so poor that, as far as many parts of your body are concerned, you're holding your breath. That's not healthy.

The next biggest factor is improving muscle strength. If your muscles are weak, the only thing handling the stress is the joint surface and that was not built for the kind of beating it takes without proper muscle support. It has been well demonstrated that by improving the muscles around the knee you can improve the internal structures by taking pressure off of them.

Sometimes when you are in pain one position feels better than others. Generally this is because you're taking pressure off of the sore spot. Muscles that are weak and flaccid can't take the pressure off joint surfaces like a muscle that's strong and taut.

By losing excess weight and strengthening your muscles, you can lessen knee pain to the point where a less aggressive rehabilitative or surgical approach is necessary. If surgery is required, the odds of success are greater and the postoperative response will be improved: casts fit better, braces fit better, crutches are easier to handle, and general mobilization is a lot easier.

REHABILITATIVE EXERCISES

Whether you've had surgery or not, establishing pain-free range of motion is first on the rehab agenda. Like the bracing, such movement facilitates healing and prepares the muscles for the next phase, reestablishing muscle strength. Static exercise is generally first, which means exercise performed without producing joint motion. This can be as simple as alternately tightening and then relaxing the musculature of your leg. This isometric exercise quickly evolves into something called the Drake seven-count straight-leg raise: (1) Your best bet is to sit on the floor, back against the wall and leaning against a pillow, which fills in the area between the small of your back and the wall. You start with a simple isometric tightening of the muscles of your leg, keeping your muscles tightened for the entire exercise. (2) You then try to pull your leg muscles even tighter. (3) Next, while keeping all of this tension, you raise your entire leg four inches off the floor and hold it there. (4) This is not a competition, so there is no count. You keep your leg up only long enough to check and make sure that none of the tension you had in your leg was lost in the raising of your leg. (5) Still without losing any of the tension, you then lower your leg back to the floor. (6) One last time you try to pull the muscles in your leg even tighter. (7) Finally, it's time to relax before trying it again. The goal is two sets performed ten times, with a sixty-second rest between sets.

This particular exercise is at first done to tolerance. Again, you're not racing with the clock; the only time element involved is the sixty-second rest between sets. If you find it impossible to keep the muscles tight throughout the exercise, then muscles should be tightened as much as possible.

After finally progressing to three sets of ten, a program of progressive resistance exercise is begun. One of the most famous trainers in the early days of sports medicine was Milo of Croton. By the fifth century, B.C., the trainer-coach had become a significant force in the development of athletics and Milo was a six-time Olympic champion wrestler. One of his training methods was to start lifting a bull on the day of its birth; by doing this daily one could lift the animal when it was full grown. This is probably the first record of progressive resistance exercise. Bulls at birth are probably still too heavy for recovering knee-injury patients, but the same principle applies: Strength comes from graduated weight work, first with ankle weights and then with more complex equipment.

In all of these exercises your goal is to bring your injured leg up to par with your uninjured leg. Try exercises first on your uninjured leg, then work toward achieving the same *quality* as well as quantity of exercise with your rehabilitative efforts. That is, if you can do exercises with your good leg without trembling, your recovering leg should manage the same quality movements. (Of course if you can't do exercises with your "good" leg without quivering and shaking, you need to rehab that leg too!)

Two simple exercises may also be appropriate once strength begins to return. One requires a single step and the other an out-of-doors. The lateral step-up routine is just what its name implies: sidestepping up a slight elevation, which helps build the thigh muscles. However, you must be ready for this exercise. Before you start make sure you can tighten your thigh muscles and lift your leg about six inches. (Sit on the floor with your back against a wall for support.) Once you can do this comfortably, without your leg quivering and shaking, for ten quick repetitions, then you're probably ready for some stair work.

Another way to help strengthen the quadriceps muscles is to hike hills. This comes after stair walking and after walking on the flat. Like any exercise, if it causes pain that causes you to stop or just makes you wish you could, then STOP. If your muscles are not yet up to hills, they won't be able to take the strain and something else will have to. That something else is the joint surface of your knee, and if you're recovering from a knee problem, the last thing you need is to overstress it. Both stair climbing and hill hiking place a lot of pressure across the kneecap area, and if you have significant areas of chondromalacia, or softening of the patellar surface, either activity can aggravate it further. So if hills cause pain, then go back to hiking along the flatlands. If stairs cause you to grimace, work on your leg lifts some more. Don't ever just stop and give up. Retreat just a few steps and recover.

In the early stages of rehabilitation, where the intensity is low, daily sessions are helpful. Once your intensity increases, however, three times a week is best. I've seen patients who figure that if I ask them for three days of exercise a week, they'll do six days a week and get better twice as fast. I've also seen these same patients return in a big hurry when they've injured themselves.

Once you're on your way toward reestablishing muscular strength, endurance is next. This is achieved through some repetitive exercise such as running or swimming or a combination of these in the form of jogging in a pool. Then comes a return of speed, coordination, agility, and power. All of these are achieved through sports-specific activities, although early in rehabilitation the activity is actually performed by means of special exercises and equipment that simulate specific sports-related movements. Later the patient will graduate to drills, practice, and competition.

Everyone wants to know "When will I recover?" It's hard for any physician or therapist to give absolute dates. With surgery we can generally predict that symptoms will noticeably decrease, function will improve considerably, and knee confidence will return consistently with every succeeding three-month interval. Approximately twelve months are required for maximum rehabilitation, but even that is just a guesstimate that will be correct for only about 60 percent of surgical knee patients. The rest may have returned to athletic participation, but they recognize that their knee function isn't better than 90 percent of their preinjury status yet. For the least complex, nonsurgical injuries, rehabilitation can be expected to take two months from the beginning of therapy. However, it is not at all unusual for more complicated cases to require three to six months.

PHYSICAL THERAPY

Although rehabilitation may be achieved with minimal input from a physical therapist, the advantage of going to a therapist is that they help teach you to see the overall pattern. While it is true that some people can guide their own rehabilitation at a well-equipped health club, the only thing worse than an unthinking therapist is an unthinking machine. At least a therapist can let you know that when you experience a certain level of discomfort, then you need to back off to a slightly lower level of activity. They can interpret pain and let you know which activities need careful monitoring and which pains are to be expected given the circumstances. They also have a variety of technologies available to help you if you're having problems recovering.

For years physical therapy (PT) was basically shake 'n' bake:

massage and whirlpools. Today physical therapists are body mechanics. They handle everything from minor repair work to major
overhauls and they do it with an array of high-technology that
would have been incomprehensible just a few years ago.

Massage, Whirlpools, and Ultrasound

Massage acts as a "mechanical cleanser," helping the body rid
itself of toxins and wastes, heightens tissue nutrition and metabolism, and helps lessen inflammation, swelling, and pain. It is appropriate for muscles surrounding an injury site; these support groups
are often weakened and irritated by injury. (NOTE: Certain medical
conditions may be worsened by manipulation, including infections,
acute inflammation, or acute bouts of arthritis, synovitis, or phlebi-
tis. If you have varicose veins, massage may also be ill advised since
if there is a blood clot, it could be dislodged. And massage may be
inappropriate at a point of acute or chronic pain.)

Whirlpools are medical Jacuzzis. They're sometimes used for
strains and sprains and after some arthoscopic procedures, although
for the latter the patient must wait several days for the surgical
portals to heal. A whirlpool bath offers many of the same advantages as massage, in addition to warming tissue more thoroughly.

Ultrasound has been hailed for its ability to transfer penetrating
heat deep into the body. The sound waves produce movement of
molecules, which gives a sensation of heat. While ultrasound does
tend to soften muscle tissue deep inside the body, it really offers
little more than other heating elements such as whirlpools.

Everyone loves shaking and baking. Patients love it because they
don't have to do a thing but sit or lie there. Therapists love it
because it's easy to do, it pays the bills, and it makes the patient
feel more comfortable. The last factor is obviously the only one of
any therapeutic importance, but you should be aware of the others
since these modalities are often overemphasized and that's what is
behind their popularity. As a painkiller, heat and massage may
manage to increase your comfort level enough that you'll do better
when it comes time for the exercises and activities associated with
your real physical therapy. But as far as mechanically or physically
altering your condition, this approach has very little to offer.

TENS, EMS, and Biofeedback

Electromedicine has become a popular—and confusing—area of

medical research. These three technologies are sometimes used in physical therapy and, like shaking and baking, are often given a little more emphasis than they deserve.

Transcutaneous electrical nerve stimulation (TENS) is derived from some of the theories of acupuncture. In physical therapy, TENS is used to promote early mobilization and allow for more active physiotherapy. It blocks pain by delivering a pulsating electric current directly to the pain site. Basically, it confuses the brain. If you've got a headache and you hit your thumb with a hammer, you may find the throbbing of your thumb drowns out your headache. TENS utilizes the same principle; your brain can manage only a certain level of stimulation.

The most appropriate candidate for TENS is someone who has been on a lot of pain medication, has grown resistant to standard analgesics, and now needs a little extra pain relief in order to get started on a program of rehabilitation.

Electrical Muscle Stimulation (EMS), or Transcutaneous Muscle Stimulation (TMS), has been proposed as a method of curbing muscle atrophy following surgery. We're not sure how this works (if it does) but the current concept behind electrotherapy is that it reduces some of the negative cellular changes that take place after surgery. EMS does not prevent muscle atrophy, but there is some evidence that it may slow down the process. Unfortunately, inconsistent and conflicting studies suggest that we're not yet ready to call this a major new therapeutic tool.

I use EMS, but not as a therapy in and of itself. Electrical stimulation gets muscles firing and functioning and literally helps patients find their muscles. Once EMS gets a muscle contracting the patient can find that muscle or muscle group themselves and start working on them with various exercises.

Biofeedback can be used the same way. We place little electrodes superficially on the skin, and when the electricity is turned on an audio readout allows the patient to hear his or her muscles contracting. As the muscles are tightened further the sound increases and again the patient is helped to find and isolate those muscles so that they can enter into rehabilitation.

There are two types of patients who may need help finding their own muscles: the patient who has never been on any kind of exercise program before and the multisurgery patient. The former need additional help isolating muscle groups simply because they've never done anything like this before. The latter have been under the knife so often that they've simply lost much of their ability to discriminate one muscle group from another.

All of these approaches are meant to do nothing more than get patients over a hurdle, move them on to the next plateau where they can exercise harder and have more control over their own therapy. I recommend these approaches for probably 10 percent of my patients. At other clinics they're prescribed much more frequently. If someone recommends one of these modalities, ask why. Never forget that there is a reward system in medicine. The medical rationale sometimes seems to be "If it helps some people and I'm getting paid to do it, then why not try it on all people and everyone will pay me to do it." Think about that: Why spend your time and effort trying to comply with the EMS instructions when you could be lifting weights and getting through therapy faster? Keep your $35 to $55 a session and take the most direct course to recovery instead of all these sidesteps that are not really therapeutic.

Cybex

With a Cybex doctors can precisely determine your muscular condition and assess whether or not you're really ready to go back to work or play. The Cybex is the electrocardiograph of orthopedics; it objectively measures range of motion, strength, power, and endurance. Unlike the dead weight of other exercise equipment, the Cybex provides isokinetic exercise, that is, it matches patient resistance: As hard as you push, it pushes back. The Cybex can also record exact capabilities on a computer. The resulting printout can compare an injured joint with an uninjured one, demonstrate therapeutic progress (or lack thereof), and point out which patients are wasting my time and theirs. It can also be used diagnostically to reveal unrecognized muscle weakness. If we find a tremendous amount of muscle weakness, maybe we need to concentrate on a strengthening program and stop looking for a mechanical problem. If surgery is imminent, the Cybex might suggest that we build up at lest some of the muscles before we even schedule time in the operating room.

Weight Training

If you do not have an exercise machine available to you, you can use weighted shoes, ankle weights, or even a purse with weights. (It needs to be a strap model.) And if none of those are available, try the sand-in-a-sock trick. Place some sand in a sandwich bag, close the bag, and insert it into a sock, which you then can drape over your ankle. Just make sure that the weights you use are not so heavy that they place stress on your knee. If you experience pain in or around your kneecap, the weights are too heavy. Also, the angle of the knee when beginning the movement should be 145 degrees or more, as measured from the back of the thigh to the back of the shin. If your leg is too far back and your shin too close to your thigh, there is too much stress placed on the knee joint at the start of the extension movement. You might be safe (but pained) with light weights, but heavy weights with that kind of flexion can actually be damaging.

Although athletes usually do well with weight therapy, sometimes they do too well. Postinjury rehabilitation is often a traumatic time for sidelined athletes. They fear for their active lives. So some tend to be overzealous, and on land this can quickly turn good intentions into muscle fatigue. What happens, we think, is that gravity resistance machines tend to overuse isolated muscle groups and neglect their opposing counterparts. Water workouts are wonderful for such patients because it's a three-dimensional resistance medium, which concurrently works opposing muscles.

Swimming

Yes, swimming. Water workouts are the new wave in physical therapy. Water is an ideal medium for therapy because it makes your body almost weightless. There's little pull on sore or deformed joints and your range of motion is considerably greater than on dry dock. Yet the active resistance of the water strengthens and tones your muscles. Compared to a regular therapy session, some people find that they almost float through tough workouts when they're doing them in water. But that doesn't mean they're not doing real work. Water running, for example, is so effective that some world-class runners use it even when they're not injured because it provides a comparable workout without the stress of gravity.

Since the buoyant effect of water eliminates impact, it is an ideal

therapy for people suffering overuse syndromes. The soothing nature of water may also distract patients from pain. And athletes
regain their sense of balance and muscle memory when they train
in a nongravity environment.

Water workouts also help you find muscle groups you might
otherwise have problems isolating, and you can work on technique
since the slow-motion effect of water workouts helps reveal movement patterns that would not be as visible on dry land. I recommend swimming to about 30 percent of my patients. It's best used
later in the rehab process when weights would be appropriate. One
problem is that when doing kicks, the greatest pressure is just when
you're starting to move your leg. When we use weight machines,
they are specially built to provide the least resistance at the start of
movement, which is a lot easier on the joint surface. As you bend
your leg the weight increases as your muscles become more capable of providing critical support.

Water workouts can also be very helpful for patients who are
having trouble getting started on weights or who have a back
condition that makes regular workouts a bit of a pain.

To get the most from your water workouts, wear fins when
swimming. They really exercise the thigh and buttock muscles, yet
you hardly ever move your knee. You also might consider wearing
tennis shoes whenever you're working out in a pool. It looks pretty
strange, but they increase resistance and improve stability during
water routines. Forget bathing suits with padded bras and skirts—
they add to your buoyancy and make your footing less secure.

So much for liquid assets, how about drawbacks? Well, you have
to have a pool, and it should have guardrails, steps, and a good
heating system. It also should have a uniform depth that allows you
to keep your head above water. Finally, there are vanity problems
such as hair and nails. Don't laugh. If it's important to the patient,
then doctors and therapists had better consider it a real factor.

For all the high-technology and expensive rehab centers, the
heart of physical therapy is still exercise. We've already discussed
some of the more common exercise routines. Now it's time to get
down to what many people think of first when they think of
physical therapy: pain.

Pain

We all know the story of the princess and the pea. The poor girl couldn't fall asleep atop twenty mattresses because a single pea had been slipped beneath the bottom one. This fairy tale is only an exaggeration of a real medical dilemma: Some people are terribly distressed by the same pain that goes barely noticed by another person.

If you have a problem with pain, consider first your personal history. Does pain generally get you down or do you belong to the "Pain? What pain?" school of masochism. If pain and you have never been on easy terms, are you doing what you can to ease your pain? Are you on any recommended medication? If you are, have you been taking it? Are you paying too much attention to your pain? Paying attention to pain makes it worse while distracting your attention lessens discomfort. Are you nervous, anxious, or otherwise in the mood to let pain get you down? If so, this may account for some of your painful response. On the other hand, if you haven't listened to pain yet in your life, this is not the time to turn a deaf ear to your body talk. Studies suggest that *osteoarthritis can be irreversibly triggered in just one poor rehabilitation treatment session.* Now is not the time to ignore pain. Contrary to what you may have heard, the initials P.T. stand for physical therapy, not physical torture.

Doctors have every right to worry about patients undergoing physical therapy. To put it bluntly, bad rehabilitation therapy is much too common. Part of the problem is the patient, part of the problem is the therapist. The "no pain, no gain" credo has no place in physical therapy. If exercise produces pain, strength is not improved, it is decreased. The risk of injury is also great when activity produces pain.

Yet it's amazing what a patient will do because a doctor, a therapist, or the guy next to them at the gym told them to do it. "Sure it hurts, and there's pain, and it's killing me, but I was told to do it, so it must be good." White coats and beepers do not perfection make. If something isn't working because there's pain, tell us, for God's sake!

But (and you knew there had to be a "but," didn't you?) discomfort is to be expected. How can you tell the difference? If, after a workout, your muscles are sore, burning, or aching, that's something you can work through, and slowly develop strength with, despite such discomfort. If an hour after therapy you have an increase in pain, an increase in tissue temperature, swelling, and a decrease in functional level, these are obvious signs you are over-doing it. Don't stop, but drop back a level and see if you're not in better shape going a little slower.

You may find you're most uncomfortable in the morning. After a night's sleep you wake up with considerable pain and difficulty walking. If you're scheduled for another therapy session that same day, you should reschedule and allow time for your tissues to rest. If you have any rehabilitation at all on a day like this, you should limit it to something simple such as whirlpools or massage.

Basically, you should not come out of a physical therapy session vibrating like a just-struck gong. If you are consistently advised to take pain medicine *before* therapy, something is wrong and odds are it's not you. When I send patients to a physical therapist I tell them if it causes a lot of pain I want them to stop whatever it is they're doing. Likewise, if they feel nothing after a therapy session except a certain lightness to their wallet, they may also have a problem. Pain is out but sweat is very much in. You're going to have to work at getting better, and that means you should expect a few sore, aching muscles.

There is one particular problem that can be extremely painful, but here, too, there is an alternative. Sometimes healing occurs with considerable internal scarring. With ligament surgery and fractures, it probably occurs 1 to 5 percent of the time. It used to be a lot more common in the days when we slapped a cast on everything. These adhesions sometimes limit flexibility and must be broken up. In the past—and all too often in the present—scar tissue or adhesions were broken up by something called a closed manipulation. The sensation is of basic body physics being horribly violated. The procedure is sometimes done in a padded room—which muffles piercing screams—other times under anesthesia. What we ended up doing with these patients was cranking on them, jumping on them, forcing the joint. When we did this there were terrible crunching sounds, and I always asked myself, "What the heck is crunching?" Was it the scar tissue breaking up or the bone surface fracturing? My professors always told us to do an X ray immediately after a manipulation to make sure we hadn't broken anything. At a certain point you ask yourself, "Isn't this a bit barbaric?"

So in 1981 my partners and I began using arthroscopy to visualize the scar tissue and then cut it out so that the limb would move more freely. Many specialists now offer this alternative, but a lot of surgeons still use the old crank approach. It's quicker and a lot simpler than arthroscopy, but you really have to hear only one manipulation to appreciate the difference. If someone told me I needed a closed manipulation, I'd ask about alternatives, and if none were offered, I'd go find someone who could offer them.

Finally, there are two types of patients who really scare me: the dead fish who just lie there and the 150 percenters. Doctors tend to relate better to the 150 percenters than the piece of lox, but both ends of the spectrum are killers.

If you ever have any question about what is or is not an appropriate level of discomfort, talk with your doctor. *Don't* just give up. I suspect that millions of people have significantly altered their lifestyles and regret having lost some of the joy from their lives due to one knee problem or another. Their true situation has less to do with losing their abilities due to injury, however, than it does with never having been sufficiently or appropriately rehabilitated. Most people would pay dearly to bring back the freedom of movement and play that they once enjoyed, but you can't just write out a check and buy back your past. You *can* work at it, and the rewards from this kind of effort may be far superior to any paycheck you've ever received.

REHABILITATION TIPS

● Early rehabilitative warm-up can include whirlpool, heating pad, or hot tub. (Note that you may have to avoid water in order to prevent infection immediately following surgical procedures.)

● Initial daily exercise routines should evolve into workouts that are done either three or four times a week.

● You should be comfortable at a particular level of therapy for at least three sessions before you increase your exercise load.

- *Even a simple exercise, done too often, can induce injury.*

- Exercise-induced joint pain, joint swelling, or prolonged muscle soreness after a rehabilitative workout suggests excessive exercise loads. Work, don't overwork.

- If you experience pain in or around your kneecap during weight lifting, your weights are too heavy.

- Rest and relax muscles between exercise sets.

- SWEAT!

15

Support Your Knee
(or It Won't Support You)

Braces and wraps have had erratic support through the years. Some professionals swear by them, others swear at them. Support runs from entire teams that use special knee braces as part of their official uniform to "all-purpose" commercial braces that experts contend could more accurately be packaged as "no-purpose" elastic wraps. If you're looking to shore up your troubled knees, there's a lot you need to know to secure real support and avoid the protection racket.

Although knee injuries have been around since the first sporting event, knee bracing is relatively new. In the early sixties most experts believed there was no way to brace a wobbly knee and stabilize it. Of course the early braces did little to reduce the skepticism. They were big cumbersome things that tended to slip out of place and fall down the leg. Then came that wonder of science, Velcro, and suddenly the knee had a real friend.

Braces didn't really find a firm place in sports, however, until 1969 when New York Jets quarterback Joe Namath had a brace designed especially for him: the Lenox Hill derotation brace. This was the first orthotic device to offer reliable protection against reinjury. Nearly half of all athletes with chronic knee instabilities caused by ligamentous damage return to their previous level of activity with the brace. Today over twenty companies are in business to brace up America's troubled knees and they offer a myriad of designs, but they all work on the same basic principles. Various stops or wedges are built into functional braces in order to prevent the leg from being completely straightened, thus preventing that last couple of degrees of extension that can cause instability. Doctors used to perform operations, called tenodesis, that would prevent the knee from going into full extension. Now braces are doing that job.

Before we review some of these devices, brace yourself: While it would be nice to be able to offer some firm supportive guidelines, there are no hard and fast rules. There is no ideal brace marketed. If there were, we wouldn't be seeing three or four new ones introduced each year. So for all the hoopla heard about braces, especially within the sports community, remember that they are just one contributing factor to knee health and happiness.

There are three types of braces: functional, rehabilitative, and prophylactic. Some people would add a fourth to that list: wraps.

FUNCTIONAL BRACE

Functional braces are individually prescribed. I tend to brace patients, particularly after an anterior cruciate ligament reconstruction, for the first year. The benefit of such bracing hasn't really been proved. I think I am protecting underlying tissue and making the brace handle some of the stresses that a functioning ACL would have handled. However, the scientist in me questions all actions and I sometimes wonder if all I'm really doing is just anchoring that knee and making the patient aware and more protective of it.

Unfortunately, despite their name, these braces aren't all that functional. For a specific event such as a football game or a ski run, they're fine, but they're not exactly something you'd want to wander through your day wearing. Because they are heavy and restrictive, you're not likely to see them on runners or receivers in football, but you may find them on tackles or drop-back quarterbacks. Likewise, in basketball, they're very good for centers or forwards, but not for guards, who have to maneuver all over the place.

Despite the competition, the Lenox Hill brace still holds about three fourths of the functional brace market. At just under two pounds, it has seven straps and, as you might imagine, it takes a little practice to learn how to hook it up properly. There are thigh and calf straps, which are common to all functional braces; two small elastic straps encircle the patella and offer kneecap support; one strap goes straight across the back of the leg and this offers critical posterior cruciate support; and two elastic straps give the brace its name by helping prevent rotation. The derotation straps start at the shin, cross behind the knee, and fasten at the thigh.

The C.Ti. is one of the lightest functional braces (fourteen to sixteen ounces) and is particularly appropriate for skiers. It even comes with an attachment so that the brace can be bolted to the ski boot. There are no derotation straps, which means you lose some protection, but there is good ACL protection and an optional patella cup can be used for posterior cruciate ligament instability. This is one of the least restrictive braces and is thus less likely to hinder athletic performance.

Functional braces are the most expensive braces available, ranging in price from $400 to $800. This price tag is largely due to the fact that each one is custom-made. Some are plastic and can be remolded if muscle bulk changes, but many are mostly steel construction, which means if the bulk of your leg changes, then the brace must be changed. If your skin is marked long after you've removed a brace, it's probably too tight or the padding needs to be replaced. Do so!

The other extreme is equally dangerous. A knee brace that is too big or too loose can do a lot of damage if the knee is struck.

REHABILITATIVE BRACES

While functional braces are shoring up some athletic careers, rehabilitative braces are saving some people from long, debilitating casting. Within the last ten years rehabilitative braces have largely replaced casts. The idea behind casting was complete immobilization to facilitate healing. Great theory, lousy practice. A tremendous amount of atrophy occurs with disuse. The key to controlling muscle atrophy is movement, so braces have been developed that allow ten to thirty degrees of knee movement. There's no severe pain, you're not in danger of pulling anything apart, and there's no threat to any tissue, yet this little jog of movement is enough to maintain some muscle function, maintain proper bone and tissue metabolism, and prevent the adhesions and stiffness that result from complete immobilization. Complete casting is now most appropriately used for fractures, although braces are being developed even for fractures.

Today's braces also allow for adjustments throughout the healing process, which means your range of motion can be increased as you heal.

Rehabilitative braces are sometimes used for rheumatoid arthritis patients, postsurgical patients, and for some post-traumatic injury patients.

Rehabilitative bracing can also be valuable if you are participating in running sports while recovering from tendinitis. The brace keeps irritation down to a minimum.

Sometimes braces are used without a clear physiological purpose. If you've been injured, a brace will remind you to take it easy. However, just because there's a bumper on your car doesn't mean an accident won't cause major damage. We've shown that most people who have been injured have residual muscle weakness because they were never sufficiently rehabilitated, and that is the key to injury prevention, not a brace. Of all the "weak knees" out there that are braced, I'd say half of them are being braced because of ligamentous damage or internal derangement and the other half are being braced merely because there's muscle weakness. If the problem is muscular weakness, the answer certainly isn't a brace. You must build your power and endurance.

PROPHYLACTIC BRACES

The third major type of brace is the prophylactic braces—braces worn to prevent injury to healthy knees or reinjury to once-hurt knees. When a player is hit from the outside this brace distributes the blow above and below the knee. Again, the theory makes a lot of sense. The problem is that while many coaches say these braces work, recent studies offer little support for their use. In a three-year study of over seventy U.S. collegiate teams reported in the January

1987 issue of the *The Journal of Bone and Joint Surgery*, researchers found preventive knee bracing may not be preventive at all and may in fact be harmful. Dr. Carol Teitz, who supervised the research project, reported that "players who wore braces had a significantly higher rate of [knee] injury than players who did not, 9.4 percent [compared] to 6.4 percent."

As a result, the NFL Players Association, which has been pushing for mandating braces, backed away from its stand. Meanwhile, several NFL coaches who in the past have unilaterally required braces are reconsidering their position.

Dan Henning, offensive coach of the Washington Redskins and director of the NFL's most comprehensive study of knee braces back when he coached the Atlanta Falcons, told the *Los Angeles Times* (April 11, 1987), "The problem with [knee-brace] research is that it is necessarily always incomplete. That's because there's no statistical way to measure the number of knee injuries *prevented* by bracing." He said that his Atlanta research showed that bracing lowered the knee-injury rate.

This debate becomes even more heated due to three major factors: risk, money, and big money. Knee injury is one of the biggest risks facing players in sports. In football alone players face about a 20 percent chance of knee injury each season and a 60 percent chance of knee injury in a four-year career. The money involved in trying to prevent these injuries is significant. When you add up the cost of the brace, taping supplies, and trainers' time, the cost of bracing is approximately $400 per player per season. But the big money comes under what I call damned-if-you-do, damned-if-you-don't litigation. In the past injured students could sue if they played for coaches who did not mandate braces. Now they may sue if they are forced to wear a brace, based on the data provided by Teitz's study.

One of my concerns about bracing is that it could provide a false sense of security: braces cannot replace strength and balance in the lower body. Alex Gibbs, a line coach for the Denver Broncos, says, "The [knee] injuries we've had were caused by imbalances—by guys who had developed the front muscles at the expense of the others." Indeed, if your limbs and muscles are not strong, any bracing is likely to fail.

If you have a decision to make about bracing, ask the coach and your physician for advice. There are two prophylactic braces that are most commonly used today: the McDavid Knee Guard and the Anderson Knee Stabler. The McDavid brace is pulled over or wrapped around the knee and secured by double Velcro strips both above and below the knee. A hinged splint bridges the upper and lower leg and acts almost like a second medial collateral ligament. The Anderson/Stabler (named after the man who invented the device and quarterback Ken Stabler, for whom the device was invented) has a pivot hinge, which may allow slightly more flexibility, and a steel-reinforced bridge, which may take more stress than plastic. Both cost about $70.

WRAPS

What about over-the-counter elastic knee wraps? These probably remind you that you have a knee problem, they may limit your movement a little, slow you down a bit, and afford you some comfort and warmth. I've worn these wraps myself and they made me feel better, but I'm not really sure why. They can't provide any real ligamentous support. But they can provide compression. Remember what we said about muscle strength diminishing pain because it "takes the pressure off" a painful joint? Likewise, when you're in pain one position often feels better than another; again, in the most comfortable position you are probably relieving that pressure.

Sometimes a wrap is used by a physician to keep swelling down. You should not self-prescribe a wrap for this purpose. This treats a symptom, not the cause of your problem; diagnosing the cause will require medical advice (from a doctor, not from the "specialist" you see in the mirror every morning).

Problems arise when any wrap or brace irritates the skin; besides abrasive irritation, additional perspiration can cause a rash. Or you can get a wrap or brace that's too tight. I have patients come to me complaining that their feet are swollen. I ask them why they are using their brace as a tourniquet.

Some people wear a brace or a wrap instead of getting their condition taken care of medically. Knee supports are useful, but they're no substitute for rehabilitation and recovery. They can help you perform specific athletic tasks, but they won't let you carry on as though you were never injured; that's especially true once you're off the field or away from the game.

In summary, there may be a place for a brace, but until we know a lot more about their impact in sports it's best to focus our attention on those factors that we know are important.

16
Arthritis Relief

We've discussed how frustrating arthritis is for both patient and researcher. People put off seeing a doctor for an average of four years after the first symptoms, largely because they think there's little that can be done for them, and researchers have still failed to come to a clear understanding of the causes for the leading chronic illness in America. But not understanding the origins of the two leading arthritic illnesses does not mean there's nothing that can be done. True, there is no "cure" yet for arthritis, but despite all the hoopla, the expensive technologies and fancy procedures, there is no cure for heart disease yet either—but for both heart disease and arthritis no one can dispute the fact that we are miles ahead of where we used to be in treatment.

So while we still have no cure, the implications of what we have learned about arthritis are significant: We now are more capable of early detection, planning appropriate management, arresting or at least slowing the disease process, and perhaps, for the first time, providing some insights that may be able to reverse the three leading causes of arthritis.

The leading causes of arthritic disability are osteoarthritis (OA), rheumatoid arthritis (RA), and gout. All three commonly affect one or both knees, as well as the hip, elbows, hands, and feet.

TREATMENT

Conservative management techniques have been greatly refined over the last few years, but, as in any disease, the earlier treatment is initiated, the more successful intervention is likely to be. Gout responds very well to drug therapy. On the other hand, RA and OA are more difficult to control. One of the best management techniques for all three forms of arthritis of the knee is maintaining proper weight. Many people with arthritis are overweight and weight reduction is essential. This is particularly true when the knee is involved, since each extra pound weighs heavily on the knee. The other key components to initial treatment include rest, exercise, and medication.

The first two of these approaches may seem contradictory, but it's more understandable if you realize that often in medicine opposites are attractive. Consider that for many injuries, one of the best therapies is the use of both heat and ice. In the case of arthritis, rest has long been a cornerstone of care, but in recent years we've come to recognize the immense value of exercise in interrupting the disease process, managing the disease, and possibly reversing it.

Rest is necessary, but rest alone may actually be hazardous to your health. Most people sleep, for example, with their knees bent throughout the night. Connective tissue, such as muscles and ligaments, will contract if not stretched occasionally. That's why everyone is a little stiff in the morning. If these tissues are inflamed, such as in the case of RA, it becomes painful to straighten the knee out in the morning. Under normal circumstances morning stiffness disappears naturally through the course of daily movement. If you want to limber up quickly, a few exercises will generally expedite the process. However, if there is pain, normal movement will be protected and it may take a while just to get your knee straightened out. Exercises are probably not the first item on your agenda since the pain would seem to preclude such exertion. Yet this results in a vicious cycle: Continued pain causes an increase in protective bending of the knee, which causes increased tightening of the tissues, which results in more pain. Eventually the knees can become flexed (bent) so badly that even walking becomes impossible. This state is called a flexion contracture.

Movement and Exercise

A key contribution of exercise is its role in weight control, which has an amazing impact on the knee. Since knees experience forces two to six times body weight during daily activities, such as walking and stair climbing, an added twenty pounds of body weight actually subjects our knees to an additional forty to 120 pounds!

Exercise also contributes to our emotional health and well-being. Looking at the psychological components of exercise in the elderly, significant improvement has been reported in morale, depression, self-concept, anxiety, and functional abilities. One study, conducted at Walter Reed Army Medical Center, Washington, D.C., examined arthritic patients who were between twenty-seven and eighty-four years old and had participated in a specially designed group exercise program. After twelve weeks the exercise group had higher morale, a more positive attitude toward their own aging, and less agitation than adults with arthritis who did not participate in such programs.

The bottom line is that exercise is as necessary to the person with arthritis as insulin and diet control are to the diabetic. Moving your body is the key to maintaining your ability to keep moving. In other words, use it or lose it.

We've seen how exercise helps keep soft tissue soft and pliable. That's one advantage. Another, which is critically important, involves how the body receives its nourishment and repairs itself. Movement transports metabolic materials through tissue, such as cartilage, and supplies the raw materials necessary for repair and maintenance. Not only does movement feed your tissues, it cleans up afterward, removing the waste products and clearing the deck for more body-building supplies. When such activity is followed by rest, tissue rehydrates itself with more of the raw materials that will start the whole process over again the next time there is exercise.

It is essential that affected joints be exercised at least once a day, even if only for a few minutes, to build strong muscles *and* increase endurance. Keep in mind that no exercises should be done that subsequently increase pain for more than an hour or two. Your exercise guidelines should be pain and swelling. If you get this kind of reaction from within the joint, back off a little on your exercise program. If you're doing twenty repetitions, back off to fifteen. But whatever you do, *don't quit!* When you cut back to zero you have taken three giant steps backward instead of one small step back. You need to progress forward, not regress and retreat.

It is best to initiate an exercise program with the guidance of your doctor and a physical therapist who can devise a program specifically for you. The amount and kind of exercise that is right for you will depend on the severity of your particular disease and the condition of your joints. Too much exercise can damage your joints and increase your pain; too little, and you give up before there's really a chance for your body to be helped by the new routine. Improvement may be slow, it may take three to six months to see noticeable improvement, but individuals who follow an exercise program closely are rewarded with easier movement.

If you're really out of shape, try starting out with five minutes of exercise twice a day. *Range-of-motion exercises* will help you regain normal joint movement. *Functional exercises* help you recover or maintain useful movements involved with daily activity. *Strengthening exercises*, such as isometrics, will increase the power or work ability of your muscles without requiring you to bend painful joints. *Stretching exercises* may be necessary if your joints won't move through normal motion because of stiffness. And *aerobic exercise* will increase your flexibility while providing all the recognized cardiovascular benefits of this kind of activity.

Range-of-Motion Exercises Range-of-motion exercises are just what they sound like: actions that put your joints through their available range of motion and, eventually, increase your range of motion. For example, you can move your leg through nearly 180 degrees of motion, but your thumb joint will probably go only ninety degrees. If you have lost some of your range of motion due to arthritis in the knee, you may have an arc of leg movement of only twenty to forty degrees or less. Increasing this arc can be as simple as raising and lowering your leg, flexing and straightening your knee, twisting—gently—at the hips.

Functional Exercises Functional exercises may have a direct impact on your daily activities. These are movements involved in doing useful things, such as performing household tasks or simple daily chores like buttoning and unbuttoning blouses or shirts. The latter may be avoided by people with arthritis in their fingers, but as we have pointed out, activity avoidance may simply compound your problem.

Strengthening Exercises Before you were injured you could exercise to get in shape. Now you have to get in shape to exercise. Arthritis can slow you down, but what it should not do, except in extreme cases, is stop you. What happens is that the pain of arthritis leads to "favoring" certain joints and this leads to muscle deterioration. In order to participate in activities such as tennis, muscles weakened by arthritis must first be strengthened.

You must strive to maintain good quadriceps strength from the moment you become aware of disease in the knee. These critical support muscles keep the knee, which is under tremendous stress in the best of circumstances, from having to support even more weight.

Start out slow and work up to ten to fifteen minutes of exercises every other day. Once you have built up your muscles, and it will take at least two months, then you can move on to more aerobic activity.

Swimming Strengtheners While swimming is a terrific aerobic exercise, the pool can be used to build up those muscles before the more vigorous activities. These strengthening exercises may be best on an alternate-day basis. Your body needs the extra time to build muscle and replenish the muscle tissues. Two good strengthening exercises are straight-leg raising and swimming with fins. (For more ideas, see the stretching and strengthening exercises in the Appendix.) In fact, swimming is a great way for you to get in shape if you have arthritis. Doing exercises in a pool or special tank (hydrotherapy) is much easier than doing them out of water. The buoyancy of the water supports 90 percent of your body weight, and the warmth of the water helps relieve pain and stiffness.

Isometric Exercises Isometric exercises are of particular importance to arthritis sufferers. If you have knee pain, try alternately tensing and relaxing the thigh muscles or repeatedly pressing the knees together. Such exercises provide a way to contract and relax muscles without requiring any real movement of inflamed joints. (See Appendix for ideas.)

There are also newer forms of exercise using specially designed exercise machines that can strengthen muscles with minimum trauma and provide a functionally better knee. These techniques are available through physical therapists or exercise physiologists.

Aerobics Now that your quads are quite strong, you're ready to begin aerobic activity, twelve to twenty minutes a day, three to five days a week. If you want to warm your muscles before moving them around (which is a good idea), try a warm bath or a long hot shower. Using an electric lamp or heating pad, a hot wet towel, or heat-inducing ointments may also help. The heat seems to slightly dilate your blood vessels and improve blood flow, carrying more oxygen to your muscles while helping carry away byproducts a little quicker.

Swimming Swimming is an excellent, low-impact aerobic activity. You can swim laps if you wish, but a walking or even running regimen in water will minimize weight-bearing or joint stress, yet still provide a good cardiovascular and strengthening exercise experience. (Many chapters and divisions of the Arthritis Foundation have special warm-water exercise programs for people with arthritis.)

Walking Walking, of course, is a good exercise, provided your knee and ankle joints are not swollen, painful, or stiff. If they are, you may have to limit your standing and walking but maintain your strength and joint motion with other forms of exercise, such as cycling or swimming.

Biking Another option is to try and pedal away arthritic pain and fatigue. Researchers at the University of Michigan School of Medicine had a group of female patients with rheumatoid arthritis pedal a stationary bicycle from fifteen to thirty-five minutes three times a week. After twelve weeks the women reported that pedaling brought them more pep and less pain and swelling. What's more, they felt that activities of daily living had become a lot easier and their interest in social activities had increased.

Ice

Although it's not as pleasant as heat, there is a place for ice in arthritis therapy. Wrapping the knee in an ice pack three times a day for twenty minutes helped twenty-four patients reduce pain and limit their need for medication during a 1981 study at Germantown

Medical Center, Philadelphia. The subjects also reported sleeping better and a greater ability to move around. In an expanded study of 274 patients, the same doctors found that 76 percent actually preferred ice packs to conventional heat therapy and 68 percent reported a preference for ice over medication.

After exercise, five to ten minutes of ice massage tends to further dilate the blood vessels, helping improve the metabolism in the area of application. For convenience and economy, freeze water in Styrofoam cups. When you peel back the top half of the Styrofoam, you have an insulated handle and an easy applicator.

Arthritis and Emotions

One of the benefits of exercise and getting your disease under control is that it helps you manage the disease emotionally. Is this important? Yes, according to some important research.

In 1985 researchers at the University of Virginia reported that as emotional stress levels increased, rheumatoid arthritis symptoms intensified and the reverse also seemed to be true—as disease activity intensified, emotional stress levels increased. The researchers concluded that identifying specific ways to decrease stress levels may, in fact, decrease the severity of arthritis itself.

Maybe this is one factor accounting for the results seen by investigators at Jefferson Medical College in Philadelphia who managed to decrease pain by tapping into the brain's own pain-relief system with hypnosis. Along with a temporary reduction in pain, distress, anxiety, and depression, there was a significant increase in blood levels of the body's natural painkiller, beta-endorphin.

Medication

The conservative management of arthritis does generally include some medication. Medication is especially important for the inflammatory diseases: rheumatoid arthritis, lupus, crystal and gouty arthritis. These are proliferative diseases of the joint lining and you have to control the disease process before you can really build strength.

In 1899 *aspirin* was found to reduce inflammation if given in higher than normal dosages. Today aspirin is still a remarkably effective drug. It not only soothes arthritis pain, but also reduces the inflammation that causes swelling and joint damage. One drawback is that it may take eight to twenty aspirin tablets a day for weeks at a time to obtain relief. In order to stomach this particular regimen, it's best to take the aspirin during meals. This may be taken literally: Midway through a meal, mix three to four tablets in with some yogurt, cottage cheese, or other food and chew. The chewing will accelerate absorption by ten to fifteen minutes and help protect your stomach lining from the aspirin assault.

In the dosages necessary for effect, some people have problems with aspirin. *Non-steroidal anti-inflammatory drugs* (NSAIDS) have become an alternative that may offer relief at lower, more convenient dosages. NSAIDS are commonly used against both rheumatoid arthritis and osteoarthritis. Names such as Motrin, Feldene, Indocin, and others are familiar to arthritis sufferers seeking pain relief. Although NSAIDS are often recommended as an alternative to aspirin, these medications also have side effects. (To learn more about the effects of various pills, see Chapter 10.)

Corticosteroids are drugs that are related to cortisone, a natural hormone produced by the body. Back about 1950 cortisone and other steroid hormones were thought to be the answer for the relief of arthritis pain. Today they may still be used briefly during acute flare-ups or on a longer-term basis for individuals with RA who do not benefit from aspirin or NSAIDS. Moreover, while oral cortisone is never used for OA, local injection of cortisone into the knee of OA as well as RA patients can be performed infrequently, and often with great benefit. It is important to realize, however, that while these drugs can provide dramatic relief, their long-term effects can also be pretty dramatic: lowered resistance to infection, stomach ulceration, cataracts, and more.

For many patients with resistant RA who have been through other drug regimens with little or diminishing benefit, there may be "gold in them thar pills." *Gold salts* have actually been used for arthritis for fifty years, but recently their use has accelerated. The problem is that it takes time to determine the correct dosage and the side effects again can be considerable. But for some patients "good as gold" can take on a whole new meaning. Once available only as a long series of injections, it was the treatment of last resort. Now oral gold is available. Besides convenience, the oral therapy also seems to have fewer side effects than injections.

One of the latest drugs to do battle with RA is an antibacterial called *sulphasalazine*, which is being touted as an alternative to gold salts. Studies in England and Scotland suggest this drug may be as effective as gold with less frequent and severe side effects.

Another potential weapon against RA is genetically engineered *interferon*, a protein that is active in the human immune system. Of the patients treated so far in very preliminary experiments at Biogen, Inc. of Cambridge, Massachusetts, two thirds reported reduced pain, swelling, and joint tenderness following treatment. The use of interferon against cancer has been the subject of considerable debate due to a long list of serious side effects. Fortunately these early studies of interferon for RA are finding results at dosages much smaller than those used against cancer. Therefore, few arthritis sufferers are reporting serious side effects from interferon.

Although a number of medications can now provide considerable relief for many arthritis patients, it's important to realize that curbing pain is a double-edged sword. Yes, you will feel better, but you must realize that the disease is still there. Pain, like death, is nature's way of saying "Slow down." On the other hand, we have seen the critical importance of continuing as much activity as possible.

Surgery

When conservative management fails and even the strongest drugs are really no match for what's going on inside the body, some form of surgery is generally the next step. For arthritis sufferers there are a number of surgical procedures that can corral the disease. While none could really be called cures, they can add more active years to life and reduce some of the debilitating pain that occasionally develops with severe arthritis. There are three main goals of arthritis surgery: to relieve pain, to correct or prevent deformity, and to improve overall movement. These goals all aim to do one thing—improve function.

Arthroscopy has introduced a new wrinkle into the surgical management of arthritis. For patients with minimal or moderately advanced osteo- or rheumatoid arthritis, arthroscopy offers a relatively safe intervention that can reduce pain in several different ways.

One arthroscopic approach is *synovectomy,* which means a surgical removal of the synovium. In rheumatoid arthritis the theory is that something goes wrong within the synovial lining of the knee joint and it becomes inflamed and starts pumping away, creating way too much synovial fluid. When the synovium is removed cells regenerate quickly and the entire lining is replaced, generally within six to twelve weeks. Perhaps 70 percent of the time the new synovium is less aggressive and without the level of disease found in the old one. Synovectomy is not a cure, but it may provide marked improvement.

The indication for a synovectomy is uncontrolled inflammation (synovitis) after six months of appropriate care. Following arthroscopic surgery the knee is sore and stiff, but infrequently are there complications.

Another surgical option is *lavage* and *debridement*. Sometimes OA patients have loose bits of cartilage in the knee that can produce inflammation. By washing out the knee (lavage), these particles can be removed and the inflammation decreased. Debridement has been compared to "mowing the lawn." Rough spots of cartilage are actually shaved and the irritating pieces whisked away by lavage. Using lavage and debridement, a long-term Canadian study of 202 knees showed an overall improvement rate of 85 percent, with 76 percent of those studied needing no further surgery by follow-up, which ranged from two to twelve years.

Lavage and debridement are not cures. If you've got a rusty hinge, you can wash it, oil it, file it down, and vacuum the floor afterward, but the hinge remains rusty, it's still damaged. Most patients like this approach because it gives them an option that is short of major surgical procedures. It will buy them time until a later date in their lives when they are less active and can undergo more major surgery.

One of those is *osteotomy,* which we have already discussed (see Chapter 5). By shifting the majority of weight-bearing forces in the knee, pain is often greatly alleviated. This procedure may allow an additional five to ten years of activity before further degenerative changes produce severe pain and functional disability. Sometimes, however, the osteotomy alone will completely avert total knee replacement.

And this is the last surgery to consider: *total knee replacement.* Although it is a satisfactory procedure, it still requires severe physical limitations and a great deal of patient cooperation in postoperative rehabilitation. (For a discussion on total knee replacement, see Chapter 13.)

Arthritis is a very frustrating disease for physician and patient alike, but there have been advances in our understanding, which now allows for more options and more relief for more patients. Like many of the problems we have discussed in this book, however, arthritis is not medically well managed without the full support and the concentrated efforts of the patient. You can't just take a pill and make it better. But you can take control of the disease—before it takes control of you.

PART THREE
Back on Track:
Safely Reentering the Active World

17

Shoes and Orthotics:
Getting to the Foot of the Matter

The feet are the foundation for the whole body. Although they comprise only a small fraction of body surface, feet exert a disproportionate influence on the rest of the body. Just try to concentrate when your feet are demanding some attention. If not treated with care and respect, feet can also cause major problems for ankles, shins, hips, back, and of course—the knees.

In the best of circumstances, the feet need support that will provide stabilization, help to absorb repetitive impacts, and protection against small and large hazards they meet while helping us move ahead. However, most feet are not perfect pieces of design and any problems affecting the knees can be multiplied several-fold when feet are called to participate in any kind of fitness program.

PRONATION / SUPINATION

If your knee hurts, you're not likely to lay the blame at the foot of your body, but that may be just where it belongs. For example, excess heel movement gets translated up your leg and can strain your Achilles' tendon or injure the cartilage in your knees. What's happening? You have excessive ankle roll, either inward (*pronation—*far and away the most common) or outward (*supination*). Lift up just the outer edge of your foot. That's pronation. Lift up just the inner side of your foot. That's supination. It's not as obvious as that when you walk or run, but if it's hurting your knee, it's more than enough. And if you suffer repeated knee problems, you may be the victim of a little too much heel movement; heel stabilization may be one solution.

Here's how to tell if you pronate or supinate: Look at a pair of well-worn shoes. If there is excessive wear on the inner surface of the heel, you travel with excessive pronation; if the wear is predominantly to the outer surface of the heel, then supination is your problem. Now look to see how your heel has held up compared to the sole beneath the ball of the foot. Pronounced wear will suggest which part of your foot strikes the ground first and thus where you need the most padding.

If your heels rock and roll, you can buy heel stabilizers or you can purchase shoes that are especially built to help you compensate for your condition. (These are available at good sports-shoe stores.) If these don't help, prescription orthotic devices might help. We'll discuss those in just a couple of pages.

HIGH ARCHES

If you have high arches, your feet are not properly absorbing shock and you may end up with either knee, shin, or lower back pain, which all suggest a need for more cushioning.

Here's a plan to check your arches. This comes from the editors of *Consumer Reports* (October 1986). Step barefoot into some water and then stand on a flat surface where your footprint can be seen. Normal feet will leave a mark an inch to an inch and a half wide at the middle of the foot. If you have high arches, the toe and heel portion of your footprint will be joined either by a thin mark or none at all. And if flat feet are your problem, most or all of the middle of your foot will leave a mark. High arches often mean a problem with supination, while flat feet are frequently associated with flexible feet that are likely to suffer from excessive pronation.

SHOES COUNT

With 300 to 400 models of running shoes alone available today, you may feel overwhelmed when you go out looking for one pair of sports shoes. Add to that a marketing industry that tends to write advertising in what one writer calls a "medical-technical Esperanto" and you have a situation so convoluted that if you can proceed with even a modicum of confidence when you walk into a shoe store, you have certainly managed a "feet" accompli. Unfortunately that knowledge is the exception, not the rule, in a country where four out of five adults complain of foot pain.

Your first order of business is selecting the proper footwear for the particular sport or activity you'll be participating in. Although they are all "tennis shoes" in the common vernacular, there are distinctly different shoes for different activities and your selection will have great bearing on your knees.

For example, let's take the simplest activity on two feet: walking. A good pair of jogging shoes could be used for walking—after all, both are forward-motion sports—but even here there are enough specific differences that if you want the best walking shoe, look for a shoe that was built for walking. Aren't they all? You've got to be kidding! Imelda Marcos could have filled several palaces with shoes and not had one comfortable walking shoe in the bunch. In fact, ladies, I am here to confirm your deepest suspicion: High heels were never meant for walking. They were popularized in the early 1500s by an Italian princess who had a squadron of servants and little more to do than watch her husband joust.

High heels throw your weight forward; that can place additional stress on knees. One of the most important functions of any shoe is cushioning, but that little point of a heel certainly is no help. And if you feel constrained in high heels, your heels agree with you. Restricted heel movement means something's gotta give, and those forces end up moving right up the leg and into the knee.

High heels are not alone, however, when it comes to being a pain in the knee. Leather soles and heels, in general, do not cushion well, yet most of the indoor world today demands well-cushioned feet, since it all seems to be nothing but linoleum, thin carpeting, or parquet over concrete. For routine daily wear the best shoe is one that is well cushioned, with a leather upper that will stretch, expand, and breathe during the day. Changing shoes during the day also allows your feet to breathe and stretch. Just as you would not feel comfortable sitting in the same position all day long, your feet would welcome a little variety. So if you have to wear more formal footwear during the business day, brown-bag more than your lunch and as soon as you're out of the office put on something sensible, something that will satisfy your very important sense of foot and knee comfort.

If you want a shoe that will support more walking than just moving around an office, for shopping perhaps or a job that requires a little more footwork, buy a shoe that is built for flexibility. A slightly elevated heel may help, since most "street" shoes have a one-inch or higher heel and a switch to flat shoes might stretch calf muscles enough to cause pain. However, high heels, no heels, and rigid heels do not permit good foot posture, especially for walking, and lead to fatigue and even injury, so these should be avoided. Again, forces that negatively affect the foot can go right up the leg and, over time, injure the knee. Even if your particular knee problem was not *caused* by foot problems, your condition can certainly be aggravated by what's happening directly south of your knees.

How to Buy Shoes

When you're shopping for shoes wear the socks or other supports you expect to use during activity. Buy shoes midday or later, not in the morning. The exception to this is if the activity you're especially buying them for is done in the morning. My co-author, for example, runs first thing in the morning. He wants his shoes to fit his morning feet, not his afternoon feet. The difference has to do with a widening and flattening of the feet throughout the day. If you had between 100 and 250 pounds or so pressing down on you, odds are that you, too, would be a little flatter after eight to ten hours.

When buying shoes make sure there is a finger's breadth between your longest toe and the end of the shoe. Most foot problems come from too tight a fit, and if your feet hurt, there's a good chance it has changed your gait or your walking style. Such changes, even minor ones, can be irritating to neighboring knees. Never buy shoes with the idea of breaking them in. Shoes should be comfortable from the first day. If your shoes are tight, you can suffer sore toes and calluses. Remember, too, that feet expand under the stress of activity. Shoes that are a little tight around your forefoot in the store can be miserable on the jogging path.

Feet also change with age. The average foot has about twenty millimeters of fat that acts as a shock absorber. As people age the amount of fat decreases and the bones in your feet become more prominent. That could lead to a greater incidence of injuries or at the very least make it easier for your feet to aggravate knee symptoms. So the older you get the more likely it is that you'll need a little extra padding in your shoes.

Although shoes are available in every price range, don't be cheap when it comes to active feet. Good shoes are worth the investment. If, for example, you're a runner and your weekly miles exceed fifteen, you should be spending at least $40 for a pair of running shoes. If you have particular problems you're hoping to protect yourself from—high arches, weak ankles, bad knee cartilage—you may have to spend even more money.

There's another reason not to skimp on protecting your feet: Most shoe companies advertise their flagship shoes and that's where their quality control is tightest. If you're buying on the low end of their shoe line, take a good look at each shoe, since it may have been stitched together with less of the sophistication, care, and high technology of more expensive models.

If you're new at all of this, throw yourself on the mercy of a salesclerk. Just make sure you're not throwing your money away. Many chain stores hire youngsters trying to work their way through school or expensive life-styles. Your best bet is a specialty store where you can talk with salespeople who participate in the same sport you do. Save a trip to the discount store for your next trip, after you have found a good shoe.

Shoes and new shoe developments occur so rapidly that it would be practically useless for us to go into specific recommendations here. The odds are pretty good that by the time you're reading this the best shoes we could mention would no longer be available, or they'd be second-best to something that's still on some manufacturer's release schedule. One piece of good news we do offer, however, is specifically aimed at women who have been frustrated in their search for active footwear.

For all their hoopla about being on the cutting edge of foot-care science, manufacturers have been slow in producing shoes of varied widths. Thus, women have been forced into either a man's shoe or a scaled-down version of a man's shoe. What's the problem? Women have unique biomechanical needs. The best known, as far as their feet are concerned, is that their feet tend to be narrower than men's feet. If women have more knee problems than men, one contributing factor certainly could be that they're wearing shoes that don't fit. Fortunately the makers of New Balance shoes seized on this foot-width difference several years ago and as we finish this book they are still the only manufacturer to offer women's shoes in three widths. Both Nike and Brooks, however, appear to be getting into the act with studies that suggest there's a bigger difference than just widths between the sexes' feet. The chief investigator of Nike's study told *Runner's World* (March 1987) that there are also proportionate differences in linear, curvature, and girth measurements of women's and men's feet. Anatomist John Robinson told *Runner's World*, "It's because of these differences that a shoe company cannot simply take a man's last [the form on which a shoe is built] and scale it down to fit a woman's foot."

A short time later Nike introduced their first poststudy model and other companies also appear to be moving toward better serving the female runner. This certainly bodes well for all women, since any doctor will tell you that wearing a shoe that doesn't fit can cause blistering, inflammation of the nerves, and, as we've noted, a variety of knee and muscle problems.

One other recently recognized difference between men and women also suggests specific advice for women shopping for shoes. Women walkers strike the ground harder than men. The Rockport Walking Institute made this discovery, and their medical director, Dr. James Rippe, speculates that women take slightly longer strides than men, which means more force when the woman's heel strikes the ground. This could be rougher on women's knees. What should women do to be able to take this difference in stride? Make sure your walking shoes are well padded at the heel.

After you've worn your shoes for a while, keep an eye on them and be ready to replace them when they show signs of wear. A study at Tulane University found that all running shoes lose about 30 percent of their shock absorbability after 500 miles of use, regardless of the brand, price, or construction. Losing that protection means you're opening yourself up to knee and leg problems, especially overuse injuries, which can be caused by excessive impact shocks.

ORTHOTICS

A good shoe won't get rid of your foot problems, but it shouldn't aggravate them either. If you are hoping to correct some inherently problematic foot features, you should think of orthotics. These are straightening or balancing devices that are very different from a simple arch support. Their main objective is to balance the foot in its neutral position throughout the walking- and running-gait cycle. While not the sole solution to foot problems, orthotics are capable of making a major contribution toward happy feet.

Orthotics are made from a cast of your foot. There are three types of appliances: soft, semiflexible, and rigid. The soft orthotics are usually made of a combination of felt and a spongy material that molds to the shape of the foot. These are often temporary inserts aimed at determining whether a custom-made orthotic is needed. The semiflexible orthotics are the most common and are often used to correct alignment problems such as pronation or supination. The rigid devices are used most often for everyday activities such as walking and are rarely used in sports because active feet can't tolerate them.

Some people would argue that there are only two kinds of orthotics—the best and the useless. Over-the-counter orthotics are available, but most professionals give little support to these shoe inserts. Their main purpose is to provide added cushioning. They may also help correct slight alignment problems. If such an orthotic proves valuable to an individual, fine, but do pay close attention to whatever problem brought you to the insert in the first place: improperly used, orthotic devices can do more harm than good. Even when used by the pros, orthotics can cause iliotibial band friction syndrome, hip and back strain, foot pain, and bursitis.

These devices can't change the shape of your foot, but they certainly can make its motion more efficient and correct certain alignment or imbalance problems. For those suffering pain in the feet, knees, hips, or back, orthotics can sometimes relieve discomfort and reduce the risk of injury.

Although a number of factors must be considered when evaluating lower extremity problems encountered by runners, a review survey done at the University of Oregon found that the records of 180 injured runners revealed that 46 percent were prescribed orthotic devices and 78 percent of these runners were able to return to their previous running programs (*American Journal of Sports Medicine* 7:6, 1979). It was also interesting that 58 percent of the runners examined exhibited pronated feet. Orthotics were able to rebalance or realign these runners' foot mechanics, take undue stress off of innocent bystanders like the knees, and return them to the pavement.

Many specialists are reporting prescribing fewer orthotics today. They just aren't as necessary with some of the newer shoes providing enough extra support and some degree of anatomic correction. Still, some sports do employ a lot of orthotic devices. In fact, so many members of the National Basketball Association use them, one trainer recalls hearing a player brag, "I faked him right out of his orthotics."

Orthotics can generally be obtained from a podiatrist or an orthopedist for $75 to $150. However, if you add in the examination, casting, X-ray and lab fees, the total cost can run to $600. Fortunately, some medical insurance plans cover them.

A FOOT NOTE

Our final thought concerns not the shoe itself but the surface it's placed upon. The relative hardness of the playing, running, or dance surface appears directly related to the potential for overuse injury. This is Public Enemy Number One as far as knees are concerned. Fortunately pain from a lower extremity overuse injury may dramatically improve by simply changing to a softer playing or running surface. Remember: Concrete and asphalt were developed for roads, not sports. While it is true that the healthiest feet are vigorous feet, there's a difference between use and abuse.

18

Conditioning:
The Road to Recovery and Prevention

On the first page of this book we noted that an estimated 50 million Americans have suffered or are suffering knee pain or injuries. Most of these pains, sprains, and strains could probably have been avoided with proper conditioning—and that's regardless of whether the injury was sports related or not. It's sad but true that too many American knees are physical wrecks waiting to happen. We are told by the President's Council on Physical Fitness and Sports that only 10 to 20 percent of the adult population exercises frequently enough and vigorously enough to meet recommended health standards. Those who are overweight or the victim of an earlier knee injury are most at risk of suffering knee problems.

If you happen to be in that group of 10 to 20 percent of all Americans who do meet the council's guidelines (at least twenty minutes of exercise three times a week, at a minimum of 60 percent of aerobic capacity), it's no cause for celebration. You have about a one in two chance of having suffered some kind of knee injury in the past, and if you did, we've seen that odds are, you were never rehabilitated. So it's quite possible that even if you happen to be in good physical shape, one or both of your knees could be so out of shape as to create a real risk of injury.

Getting the support muscles of your legs in shape is one good way to lower this risk. That means a good conditioning program.

This may sound like an exercise life sentence, but we're actually only talking about getting the leg muscles to a normal strength. Then the activities of normal living should be able to keep them up to par.

Exercises are certainly one answer, but all too often people consider exercise and activity as being synonymous. A good exercise regimen will provide overall muscular improvement. Conditioning does not mean simple activity. Individual sports tend to improve individual muscle groups. That's why a young runner may have flexible quadriceps muscles but dangerously tight hamstrings, which can be especially hazardous to the knee. All muscles come in pairs, each one balanced by another that performs an opposite function. If either the hamstrings or the quadriceps become too strong, it can cause an inordinate pull on one side of the knee joint, predisposing the knee to stress and possible injury.

If you build up the strength in your legs, that will save your knees, right? Well, not quite. The fatal flaw in too many athletic pursuits has been an overemphasis on strength training at the expense of flexibility and specificity. As muscles get stronger they tighten and so become more prone to strains and tears, much like a too taut violin string is prone to break.

If you have been a couch potato for some time, it's going to take a while to peel off all those years of inactivity. The rule of thumb is this: For a nonactive person to get into condition, it will take a month of exercising for every sedentary year. That may seem discouraging, but remember that the human machine rusts out long before it wears out. Getting into shape will never be easier but, if you wait, it could get harder. As one delightful lady who is still climbing mountains at the age of ninety puts it, "It's never too late till you're dead."

FLEXIBILITY

As we age we lose range of motion, but most of this restricted movement is due to an almost total lack of awareness of how to keep our bodies flexible. Yet you can easily stretch almost every muscle group in your body by placing your hands on the chin-up bar, thumbs facing each other, bending your knees and s-t-t-r-r-e-et-t-c-c-h-h-i-i-n-n-g-g. Although this particular approach is ideal for inactive individuals, most active youngsters and even some professional athletes could benefit from this practice.

Stretching must be part of a total warm-up regimen. At one time we felt that a little stretching beforehand would adequately prepare us for activity, but we now realize that there's a little more to it than that. We first recognized a problem when we began getting reports that adding a stretching regimen to conditioning programs did not always have positive results. Many teams and individual athletes reported an increase in muscle injuries, and runners claimed an increase in injuries as a result of stretching. What we came to understand is that stretching cold muscles can actually be quite hazardous. The individual risks suffering a painful "muscle pull." The old bouncing and bobbing "ballistic" technique certainly stretched muscles, but sometimes it would trigger "the stretch reflex": a muscle would contract suddenly against this kind of forceful resistance and, with a grimace, the athlete would feel a pulled muscle. Think of a rubber band under tension. It is suddenly lengthened and then unexpectedly, it breaks or ruptures.

Does that mean you now have to warm up to warm up? Not exactly, but it does mean that stretching alone is not an appropriate warm-up and it certainly shouldn't be the very first part. If you want to do a few minutes of exercises to get blood circulating and the body primed for activity, *then* proceed to stretching, that would be appropriate. If you're a runner, perhaps your warm-up might be several minutes of light jogging before you stop to stretch. However, a few obligatory deep knee bends and toe touches do not constitute an adequate warm-up. Your best bet is to start at the top of your body and work your way down. (See Appendix A.) Neck and shoulder exercises reduce tension in those areas. Torso exercises can limber up the back and the groin area. Lower extremity exercises are especially good preparation for activities that involve running or jumping.

None of these exercises should be done vigorously. All you want to do is increase muscle tissue temperature, which results in an increased range of motion because your muscles become more pliable and resistant to injury. At the same time you're literally getting your blood circulating. In a sedentary position the major muscles of the body receive only 12 percent of the blood supply, but during vigorous activity they require about 88 percent.

When you're ready try a static stretch, which has been shown to be just as effective as the old ballistic method for markedly improving flexibility, but it poses less risk of injury and does not cause the soreness that is often associated with ballistic stretching. Static stretches are done by bending, pushing, or pulling some part of your body slowly and gently until a stretch is felt. Hold this for five to thirty seconds, depending on the part of the body and the size of the muscles involved; the smaller the muscle set being stretched, the less time necessary to complete a good stretch. This should be repeated several times, stretching a little farther each time. Remember: Stretching should be done *slowly* and it should not be painful. In a good overall flexibility program, a routine of twelve to twenty-four "strexercises" should be used. (See Appendix A.) Once you have concluded your workout, another period of slow stretches can also be very beneficial.

Is all this really worthwhile? Well, we know that stretching the hamstring muscles, for example, can help prevent knee injuries. In particular, increasing hamstring flexibility takes some pressure off of the kneecap. Furthermore, the end-of-activity stretch has been shown to virtually eliminate postexercise muscle problems. It helps remove lactic acid, which has built up in muscles during activity, and it helps improve metabolism and stimulate blood flow, both of which assist in pain-free recovery. A warm-up also promotes agility and alertness while decreasing movement time, which means in an emergency you should be able to get out of the way faster and perhaps avoid a crash course in injury. Improving the range of motion of your joints will allow better technique, an easier acquisition of skills, and, of course, fewer injuries. Finally, warming up is relaxing, which means you're calmer and more capable of concentrating.

It is important to remember that increasing flexibility is a gradual process. If you are just beginning a stretching program, it will take several weeks before benefits occur. In fact, athletes who do not begin to stretch until the beginning of their season will receive minimal benefits, if any, that season. A year-round, daily stretching program is best, but if that's not possible, stretching should begin at least six weeks before preseason training.

STRENGTHENING

Strengthening exercises in and of themselves are very important in preventing injury, especially to the knee. Most of the protection afforded the knee comes from the powerful quadriceps muscles, their back-of-thigh neighbors, the hamstrings, and the calf muscles. These muscles control the movement of the knee. They are like the reins of a horse. If they do not have proper tension, just as a horse will wander, the control of the joint will be lost. Moreover, when these muscles are weak, the knee is not only unprotected, it has to assume a much greater load and this can be painful.

Strengthening will also increase endurance. If you suffer knee pain midway through a busy day, you are feeling an endurance problem. What do you have to do? Two simple exercises: (1) Do straight-leg raises from a sitting position; (2) while sitting with your leg straight out, tighten your leg muscles for a slow five count, then flex your leg and repeat. (See Appendix A.)

ISOMETRICS

When you use the second of the above two exercises, you are using isometrics, that is, one system of muscles contracted against another, with no appreciable joint motion. This type of exercise is often used in the knee when joint effusion makes motion painful. When using isometric exercise in the legs, remember to train the muscles in their full range of motion. In other words, if you perform isometric exercises always with the leg straight, you'll miss helping some of the muscles that go to work when the leg is being bent.

When doing isometric exercises each muscle contraction must be followed by a period of complete relaxation of sufficient duration to permit your tissues to receive an abundant supply of oxygen-rich fresh blood. (Use the "Rule of Fives": Hold the contraction for a count of five, relax for a count of five, then repeat.) If you have ever wondered why your muscles complain when you overexert, one reason is they can't "breathe." Inhale deeply. Exhale fully. Now don't breathe for about fifteen seconds. Your lungs are not pleased. They want oxygen so bad they hurt. The same holds true for your muscles: The blood comes through bringing fresh oxygen and other metabolic building blocks, and it carries away fatigue-producing waste products. (By the way, you have begun breathing again, haven't you?)

MACHINE CONDITIONING

There are a variety of weight training machines available today. They are still expensive, but many people gain access to them with a health club membership. There is nothing innately wrong with this type of equipment, but it is best used with qualified supervision. By qualified I don't mean the instructor looks good in tights—he or she had better have some specific training in exercise physiology.

Stationary rowing machines are enjoying a wave of enthusiasm right now, but like many things, there are advantages and disadvantages. They are considered to be an excellent aerobic activity—even better than the stationary bicycle because more muscle groups are used and there's more muscle strengthening going on. In contrast to jogging, rowing avoids the problems of stressed knees, hips, and feet. It places considerable load on the legs and hips, however, making it an unwise choice of exercise for anyone with an existing back problem.

CALISTHENICS, ET AL

Have you noticed something missing from all this talk about conditioning? At one time, before aerobics became a household word, exercise for many people was calisthenics. Jumping jacks, push-ups, sit-ups, and deep knee bends were the heart of any fitness program. Today they are not the exercises of choice. They don't stretch your tight muscles, don't strengthen your weak ones, and they don't even use your muscles in the same manner you will use them during athletic activity. Other than that, they had a lot to offer—for example, they were hell on knees.

Calisthenics are ballistic in nature, and we've already discussed the hazards of employing quick, jerky movements. This extreme orthopedic stress on the joints is a particular hazard to the knee. Deep knee bends, squat thrusts, "duck walking," and more have no place in a good fitness program. These are as detrimental as they are valuable. A few people still use deep knee bends, but they are modified. No longer do they dip down as far as possible. They stop about two thirds or three fourths of the way down. If you want to stay safe, imagine that there is a chair or bench underneath you and go down until your seat touches the invisible seat. If your imagination is overworked, use a real bench or chair.

Stair climbing is often touted as a great conditioning exercise, and it would be if we had knees that didn't act like they were designed by committee. Take the poorly protected knee, add the incredible forces involved in stair climbing, and you've got well-trained athletes complaining of knee pain whenever they run the stadium stairs. Even a retired security guard can give these athletes a little medical advice: Stop with the stairs already! The compressive forces on the patella are increased five times body weight when ascending the stairs and seven times body weight on the way down the stairs. Let's see, 7 times 170 pounds—that's nearly 1,200 pounds across each knee when I'm walking down a few stairs. If you'll excuse me, my knees and I will take the elevator.

We've got an appendix filled with stretches and exercises. You're really only limited by your own creativity and your body's ability to keep up with you. When you undertake your own conditioning program the following guidelines may help. Most were prepared by Dr. Bryant Stamford, director of the Exercise Physiology Laboratory at the University of Louisville, Kentucky, for *The Physician and Sportsmedicine* (13:11, 149, 1985):

1. Start from your head and work your way down your body.
2. Perform each exercise slowly, under strict control, and in perfect form.
3. Keep momentum to a minimum and never bounce.
4. Be careful when bending forward. This places tremendous stress on the lower back, especially with the knees held straight— the old-fashioned toe touch probably does more harm than good. A better hamstring stretch can be performed lying on the back and drawing the knees to the chest one at a time, with the opposite leg fully extended.

5. Exercise may cause some muscle soreness the following day
or even following the exercise program. However, if there is any
true pain, swelling, or crepitation (grating) that develops within
your knee joint, consult your physician immediately.

19
Running Scared?

The biggest trick to running is avoiding injury. When it comes to recreational injuries runners lead the pack. The annual incidence of injuries to runners ranges from 23 percent to 57 percent, depending largely on the number of miles run. Unlike most sports participants, however, runners experience very few acute injuries; instead, it is chronic stress that seems to dog almost all runners. Fortunately most of these injuries are preventable. Considering that some 30 million joggers currently run at least one mile three times a week, that's a lot of avoidable injury.

Although most nonrunners take a perverse pleasure in pointing out the hazards of running, there is no reason for joggers to be running scared. Proper risk management can make it one of the safest of all athletic endeavors.

True, running is hard on the musculoskeletal system, but the figures indicate that the body cannot only survive but thrive in the face of such activity. For a long time experts wondered whether Americans were running themselves right into osteoarthritis. Several studies have now discounted the arthritis/running link, suggesting instead that running has a protective effect against osteoarthritis. Dr. Richard Panush of the University of Florida, Gainesville, found that on a scale of 0–3 (with three being the most severe) average knee degeneration was 0.33 for nonrunners and only 0.06 for runners.

Likewise, Dr. Nancy Lane, of Stanford's Arthritis Center, discovered that bone-mineral density of runners was 40 percent higher than nonrunner's. In other words, runners have stronger bones. Even after menopause, when women's bones often become so thin that they fracture easily, the bones of female runners were denser than nonrunner's.

Indeed, a study at Children's Hospital Medical Center, Boston, found that people who run short to moderate distances (up to thirty miles a week) have no greater incidence of joint pain and eventual arthritis than people who swim, which is a sport that puts almost *no* strain on joints.

So why all the injury? Well, the two biggest problems are training irregularities and faulty biomechanics. Combined, they probably account for 80 to 90 percent of all injuries. Fortunately both are almost always correctable. The big question is: How?

BODY CHECK

Let's check your body first. If you have either knock-knee or bowleg tendencies, running is going to be especially hard on your knees. If you tend to be bowlegged, you're more susceptible to iliotibial band friction syndrome, which is a particularly painful and all too common condition among runners in general. If knock-knees is your problem, even moderate running can play havoc with your kneecap's stability. The added stress tends to move your kneecap toward one side and it rubs against the femur, causing pain. If you have either of these problems, you still may be able to run, but you'll certainly need some assistance selecting a proper shoe and/or a shoe insert to compensate for your malaligned legs.

One good piece of biomechanical news has to do with people built at a slight tilt. There have been endless warnings in the popular press that predict dire consequences from running with even minor leg-length discrepancies. The concern is based, at least in part, on a theory that suggests that biomechanical problems are magnified threefold by the consistent pounding of running. Thus, the theory goes, a one-fourth-inch leg-length discrepancy in runners would be as important as a three-fourths-inch discrepancy in a nonathlete. However, researchers from Oklahoma Children's Memorial Hospital examined thirty-five male marathon runners and concluded that discrepancies of up to an inch (twenty-five millimeters) are not necessarily a functional deterrent to marathon runners. Furthermore, no consistent benefits could be attributed to the use of a lift.

Contrary to popular opinion, too, this survey of athletes found little difference between the incidence and amount of leg-length discrepancy in marathon runners and the population at large.

New studies suggest that some running problems are gender-related. Women tend to have more chondromalacia than men, but men (surprise) tend to have more of a problem with knee instability. This last finding (based on over ten years of data gathered as a part of an ongoing study of running injuries by Dr. Douglas Jackson and podiatrist John Pagliano) is interesting when it's recalled that women are often considered to have a greater incidence of knee instability problems. Any explanation? No one's sure, yet, but it could be that men are more likely to have suffered a previous knee injury.

You may have been born to run, but what has happened to your knees since has a direct bearing on your success or painful failure as a runner. You need to exercise extreme caution if you have a history of knee problems. Almost any knee problem can be compounded by running. This does not preclude your participation—unless your doctor specifically forbids you from running—but it does mean that you had better make sure that you follow these guidelines before you put one jogging foot outside your front door:

1. Check with your doctor and make sure you have recovered from any past knee problems.

2. Follow training guidelines carefully.

3. Unless you followed a specific rehabilitation program following your injury, now's the time to rehab your legs.

4. Your running regimen should also include a general conditioning program for your legs.

5. If your old injury should flare up, curb your running immediately and seek medical attention.

CONDITIONING

Just because your old knee problem hasn't bothered you for years doesn't mean you're home free. You may believe your knees are in great shape, take pride in the admiring glances received by your unadorned legs, and still have one (or more) dangerously weakened knee. The problem is that knee injuries heal but they can leave you with muscle deficiencies of 30 percent or more, which increases your risk of injury considerably. To check your strength, test yourself with the straight-leg raises detailed in Appendix A. You should be able to do three sets of ten repititions per leg lifting fifteen to eighteen pounds. If you find that you have problems with this routine, then start with unweighted leg lifts and build up your muscles before you start to run.

If you have access to resistance weight machines at a health club, check the power of your legs. Again, work on improving the strength of the weaker leg—unless both are equally weak, in which case it's time to put both of your legs through their muscle-building paces first before you let them loose to roam the jogging path.

Running strengthens your hamstrings (in back of your thigh) and your calf muscles, but it also tightens these muscles, which means a risk of pulled muscles or tendons. To counteract this, make sure you include a pre- and post-workout stretching program (see Appendix A) in your running routine.

In addition, you can help prevent injuries to your knees by building your thigh muscles (quadriceps), which don't get much of a workout from running. There's a double benefit here. First, if you've ever had knee problems, the quads are the first to weaken, yet if they're strong they can in and of themselves help relieve some of the pain associated with various knee conditions. Second, if you run a lot, your hamstrings become too powerful relative to your quads; only by working on your quadriceps can you correct a risky imbalance. If you need to work on building or rebuilding your quadriceps muscles, there are specific exercises for this in Appendix A.

Another way to build both the quadriceps and the hamstring muscles is to hike hills. If you have a knee problem, this could exacerbate your condition. However, if hill work doesn't cause any knee complaints, it's certainly a pleasant alternative to exercises.

SHOES

Proper footwear seems to be a significant factor in running safely. This means you shouldn't just grab an old pair of tennis shoes and go running. The real tennis shoe is built to supply good side-to-side movement for racket sports. They're heavier and stiffer than running shoes and built for stop-and-go action. Running shoes also grip the surface well, but the grip is for movement that is primarily forward.

When shopping for running shoes select a shoe with a durable, multilayer sole to absorb shock and an elevated heel to reduce stress on your Achilles' tendon. The uppers should be of a smooth material to prevent blisters.

The shoes you select should feel good the first time you have them on. If they feel bad in the store, they'll feel worse after you've come down on them a couple of thousand times during a run.

Running flats are especially light shoes that sacrifice some shock absorbent protection in favor of lightness for speed. These racing shoes should not be used for routine workouts since over time they will almost certainly maim the user.

When outfitting running feet, of particular importance is a proper balance between too much and too little heel movement. Too much foot control can aggravate symptoms, but too little can likewise cause iliotibial inflammation, runner's knee, shinsplints, and Achilles' tendinitis. These injuries are usually associated with excessive ankle roll, either inward (pronation) or outward (supination). If you want to check your own roll problem, just examine a well-worn pair of running or street shoes. Check for extra wear along either the inner (pro-) or outer (supi-) edge of the heel.

Probably the most common problem is excessive pronation. Shoes with heel stabilizers or extra arch support are two options (see Chapter 17). If these don't help, prescription orthotic devices might. Also, pay close attention to the condition of your shoes and replace them when they show marked signs of wear or a significant decline in shock absorbent ability. Generally, three to six months of use is about as much as you should try to get out of any one pair of shoes. That's assuming you run several miles several times a week. If you run only once a month, your shoes will probably last considerably longer.

TRAINING

Training irregularities are the other leading cause of injury. Most of the training errors that occur are the result of pushing too hard too fast. Problems usually arise when overly eager runners try to increase distance by more than 10 percent a week. To a point, it's not how much you do but how fast you increase distance. I say "to a point" because experienced runners will eventually find that they can go no farther or faster. So the 10 percent weekly increase in distance should be a guideline and not a hard and fast rule.

Simply put, you do not want to outpace your body's ability to keep up with you. Increased activity causes osteoclast cells to kick into action and start gobbling up bone. That may sound a bit frightening, but the osteoclasts are just part of the bone-building process and they're making way for their associates the osteoblasts who lay down newer, harder, firmer bone. When this process is complete—and we're talking three to twelve months here—the runner's bones will be strengthened. Until then, however, the osteoclasts are always out in front in this race, thus weakening the bone until the osteoblasts catch up. If the runner races ahead, so do his osteoclasts. In some cases to the point where stress will cause cracks and actual fractures.

The training errors that occur usually involve one or a combination of these seven things:

1. Training distances beyond one's capacity.
2. Rapid changes or deep increase in mileage.
3. Training technique changes (eg., going from slow, long-distance workouts to rapid, short-interval workouts).
4. Constant running on hard or uneven surfaces.
5. Inadequate or improper footwear.
6. Insufficient rest between workouts.
7. Inadequate muscle strengthening and stretching.

COMMON RUNNER'S PROBLEMS

Getting on the right track in training also means understanding the problems that most often trip up runners. By far the most common knee problem for runners is chondromalacia, a tracking abnormality of the patella frequently referred to as "runner's knee."

Chondromalacia Patella ("Runner's Knee")

Chondromalacia accounts for 25 to 40 percent of knee problems treated in running clinics around the country. (You should review the summary of this disorder in Chapter 5.) A typical patient with chondromalacia is a novice or short-distance runner who has recently increased mileage or added hills. Also, women are slightly more likely to suffer this problem than men, and runners who overpronate are also more susceptible.

When your thigh muscles are weak, injured, or just out of balance, the normal smooth action of the kneecap is disrupted and the underlying surface of the patella can become irritated. The pain is described as an aching or soreness around or under the kneecap, which is aggravated by stair climbing or hill running. There may be associated swelling after a workout, a sensation of "fullness" in the knee, and stiffness associated with sitting. Symptoms may be cyclic, with periods of no symptoms followed by flare-ups. Any attempt to "run through" this injury only makes it worse and forces medical attention.

For treatment, rest from running is essential. Although you may be able to alleviate chondromalacial pain by running with your feet turned in, or pigeon-toed, this can be done for a limited time only, and even then it places dangerous stress on other areas of your legs and knees.

Once the pain subsides and the exercise program described in Chapter 5 has been under way for a couple of weeks, you may begin a graduated program of running as long as there is no pain. (If you have a subluxation problem with your kneecap, a horseshoe brace may be worn while running.) Ice should be applied to the knee after you run and moist heat may be applied several hours later. During recovery, weight training should continue and all hills should be avoided.

Knee wraps, straps, or braces may be prescribed, although a good orthotic is probably best. A temporary orthotic device may be used as a clinical test to check for effectiveness, then a permanent one may be built if the device is successful.

Steroid injections are sometimes used to alleviate early symptoms, but this approach is not really appropriate since correcting the problem is always more beneficial than burying the symptoms.

The best preventive measure you can take is to make quadriceps strengthening exercises a regular part of your exercise routine.

Iliotibial Band Friction Syndrome

In Chapter 5 we discussed iliotibial band friction syndrome (IBFS). The iliotibial band is the bundle of hip-to-knee muscles that rub against the condyle at the outer end of the femur. The syndrome usually results from a training error—most often a rapid increase in mileage or speed, changing to a hilly terrain, or consistently running on a slanted surface (which causes a problem for the downside leg). Once the training error has been made, there is a delay until the appearance of symptoms. It takes time to trigger and sustain an inflammatory reaction from all that rubbing against the lateral femoral condyle. Often pain will start within two weeks, but the runner often ignores the pain or attributes it to some other factor. (Runners often have more theories than shoes.) Thus begins a series of home remedies that eventually end in the doctor's office.

Women may be less likely to develop iliotibial band irritation because of greater ligament laxity, less prominent lateral femoral condyles, and more subcutaneous fat than men. (In one ongoing study of over 3,000 injured runners, men with this condition outnumber women four to one.) High arches and bowlegs may predispose a runner to this injury. The typical runner with IBFS has run twenty to forty miles a week for more than one year. Most complain of pain after running a consistent distance, which ranges from one half mile to ten miles.

Pain is on the outside of the knee and it can become severe, although actual damage done to the knee is not as serious as that caused by other disorders. At the first sign of symptoms it's best to cut mileage and use ice immediately after a workout. Ice and heat increase blood flow to the area and promote healing. Once the symptoms are controlled, stretching exercises are important (see Appendix A). The tighter the iliotibial band, the more friction there will be across the lateral femoral condyle.

All of these measures are aimed at alleviating symptoms, not correcting causes. That's why researchers at the University of Cape Town Medical School in South Africa decided to see if they couldn't better identify runners at risk and direct treatment to specific caus-ative factors. To obtain more complete long-term follow-up of athletes with IBFS, they treated and then followed thirty-six long-distance runners for at least one year.

When they published their results (*The Physician and Sports-medicine*,12:5, 118+, 1984) they reported that 63 percent of the injured runners were wearing or had recently changed to a hard running shoe. Running on even a mildly sloping surface appeared to promote injury in the downside leg. However, contrary to com-mon medical belief, leg-length variations again didn't seem to be an important factor in injury.

Knee Instability

Once injured, ligaments lose much of their strength, and unless specifically rehabilitated, they will remain weakened. When these ligaments can't do their job, you're left with an unstable knee and a high risk of further injury.

There is a certain diabolical aspect to this disorder: If ignored, your unstable knee can damage your healthy knee. The problem is that if your weak knee can't carry its full load, your other knee will have to absorb extra stress.

If damage isn't severe, muscle strengthening may be all you need. If it's a severe problem, bracing or even surgery to repair ligament damage might be necessary.

If you'd like to avoid future problems, you might want to have an expert check your running to make sure you've developed a con-trolled and efficient style.

Popliteal Tendinitis, Bursitis, etc.

Pain in the back of the leg, behind the knee, is fairly common, and generally it's something called popliteal tendinitis. The poplit-eus is a flat, triangular muscle located at the back of the knee joint between the femur and the tibia. It helps to flex the knee. Popliteal tendinitis is commonly associated with downhill running or running along a beach or banked surface. Pain may begin during activity (especially downhill running) or within twenty-four hours of exten-sive walking or running. Symptoms tend to cease within forty-eight hours.

The treatment for popliteal tendinitis is the same as that for

IBFS—correction of the biomechanical problem, a change in running routine, and conservative rehabilitation measures.

Downhill running is also associated with inflammation of the pes anserinus. (Remember, we didn't name these things, we just report them.) This is actually a form of bursitis and is also found in runners who are marathon training. The pes anserinus is an ending point for several muscles just below and adjacent to the patella. There is a bursa here that becomes enraged by abuse and, like an air bag in a car, it inflates in an attempt to cushion the muscles from trauma, only in this case the inflating material is fluid, not air.

Bursitis, in general, is also a common complaint of beginning runners. They often feel they can run farther or faster than the previous day. Their knees beg to disagree. If diagnosed early enough, an ice massage after running may be helpful without restricting activity. However, if left to deteriorate, the condition is best treated with rest for three to six weeks, aspirin, and ice massage. In some particularly difficult cases some physicians report that a knee splint for four to six days will shorten rehabilitation time. A chronic problem may be alleviated with a neutral orthotic.

There are two other problems that sometimes catch up with runners: patellar tendinitis ("jumper's knee") and plica-related syndromes. Both of these problems are discussed in detail in Chapter 5.

It is important to understand that while all runners will experience some discomfort associated with their activity, pain should not be ignored, especially if it does not go away with rest or becomes worse with running. There's an attitude that implies you aren't really a runner until you've had an injury. For the compulsive runner, performing with pain is a test of character. It is also a good way to get hurt.

SEEKING MEDICAL ADVICE

If you find that you are injured, seek professional advice. Once this was complicated by the fact that physicians were not at all attuned to running and runners. Fortunately, over the last few years, more doctors have become sensitive to runners' needs. It's not as common, anymore, to find a runner complaining that he can run only half the distance he used to and a physician suggesting that he should run only half the distance he used to. This is certainly not the goal of the runner, and it shouldn't be the goal of the physician. The medical profession's effort should be aimed at allowing each runner to achieve his or her own goals, however difficult it should prove.

Many runners are better informed today, which can mean better medical communication. However, it can also mean much more confusing medical communication. When a runner brings in two grocery sacks filled with shoes, orthotics, and medications, it's not so much an examination as it is a demonstration of the runner's susceptibility to advertising. Fortunately it may be possible to do an end run around much of the merchandise by obtaining a very careful history of the runner's complaint.

Dr. Robert E. Leach, professor and chairman of the Department of Orthopedic Surgery, Boston University School of Medicine, compiled a list of questions for physicians to ask injured runners (*Sports Medicine*, 5:9, 1233+, 1982). These are the questions you should be asked, and if you're not asked, you should take the initiative and volunteer the information:

- Realizing that your pain probably developed gradually, can you pinpoint a time that you noticed the pain begin?

- Was there a change in your training pattern, increase in mileage or hills, or did you suddenly start doing interval workouts?

- When does the pain occur?

- Is it present at the beginning of a run or near the end?

- Does the pain persist or increase with running, and how is it the next day?

- Is this pain present only with running or is it associated with normal activities?

- Is there pain when going up and down stairs or ramps?

- What physical manifestations have you noticed: Swelling? Popping or grinding within the knee?

- What previous treatments have you had?

- Has there been a shoe change?

- Orthotics?

- Medications?

- Injections?

- Have exercises been prescribed, and if so, which ones?

- What has been their effect?

KNEESAVERS

If you want to save your knees and run happily ever after, keep these tips in mind:

- If you want to increase your distance, limit yourself to a mileage increase of 10 percent per week. If you add hills, decrease distance. Of course it's best to run on a soft, even surface, avoiding both downhill, sidehill, and consistent canted running.

- Hills are a lot like speed—unless you're training for a race, you really don't need either. While downhill running would seem to be a breeze, it's much riskier for joints and muscles than struggling uphill. On the downside, your stride lengthens and your weighted impact with the ground can easily double. You are also more likely to lose control, which could cause significant injury. Your distorted downhill gait can also cause "runner's knee."

- If hills absolutely must be a part of your training, zigzag down the hill with your knees bent and a slight forward lean to your body. (If you run along the road, your zigging and zagging are best done on a sidewalk to diminish your chances of becoming a hood ornament on a passing car.) If pain persists despite this downhill maneuver, try a slow and controlled walk downhill. If this eventually causes pain, too, then it's time to reroute and recover.

- If you run more than three miles a day, five days a week, you are dong it for some reason other than cardiovascular fitness. Beyond this level the cardiovascular benefits are minimal but your chance of incurring an injury rises exponentially.

- Besides strengthening of the quadriceps muscles, stretching of the hip flexors, hamstring, and adductor muscle groups is important for recovery from knee injury.

- While recovering from a knee problem, bicycling or swimming are generally good alternative activities for runners.

- Too many joggers postpone seeking help when they show signs of injury. They seek medical advice only after the injury has progressed far beyond the point where it can be easily treated. Minor pains can become major problems quickly in a runner's knee. *If you've got a problem, seek professional advice quickly.*

Although the data is certainly not all in, it would appear that if handled in a responsible and intelligent manner, running need not be as dangerous as the statistics suggest. Indeed, it could actually be safer than many other activities. However, safety, like good health, takes time and attention. Take the time, pay attention, and reap the benefits of running.

20

Aerobics:
The Dance of the Injured Knee

According to the *American Journal of Sports Medicine*, aerobic dance is currently the largest organized fitness activity primarily for women in the United States. Ten years ago, when the aerobics boom blasted off, no one guessed that an estimated 25 million people would eventually be jumping, hopping, and running in place to a pulsing musical beat. Likewise, who would have suspected that something offering this much fun and fitness would cause such medical controversy? Many studies have attempted to document the hazards of aerobics. The injury rate most often quoted by the popular press was based on one California doctor's study of 1,233 students and 58 instructors. In 1985 he reported a 43 percent injury rate for students and a 76 percent rate for instructors. Apparently never have so many been so fit in such pain. However, it's good to remember that breathless statistics are often more hot air than fact.

Just how dangerous is aerobic dance? The Center for Sports Medicine in San Francisco set out to determine the injury rates for aerobic dance in order to compare it with other sport or fitness activities. Detailed questionnaires were filled out by 351 students and 60 instructors and then followed up by weekly phone calls for sixteen weeks in order to gauge participant activity levels and medical complaints. Their overall rate of injury was 44.1 percent for students and 75 percent for instructors. Although this echoes previous estimates of injury rates, the authors of this study point out that the figures are pretty meaningless: Three fourths of the "injuries" could be better described as "complaints." These participants indicated that their "injuries" were mostly muscle aches or strains that resulted in no disability. Furthermore, nearly 20 percent of the remaining injuries resulted only in an interruption of aerobic activity, but no alteration of normal activities. That left only about 5 percent of the injuries affecting daily activity and only about 2 percent requiring medical attention.

Why are instructors at such apparent risk of injury? Primarily because the time they spend doing aerobics is so much greater. When the rate of injury is compared to hours at risk, instructors have fewer injuries per hour than students.

According to the same study (*American Journal of Sports Medicine,* [14:1, 67+, 1986]), foot and shin/leg complaints were the biggest problem for students and instructors alike. Knees were next in line with students, but ankle problems inched past the knee for instructors.

BODY CHECK

One important statistic from the San Francisco study concerns students with previous orthopedic injury. If there was a history of foot, ankle, knee, or shin/leg injury, the participants were at least twice as likely to sustain similar injuries as compared to their previously noninjured counterparts. The authors concluded that it would be prudent to provide extra instructions or cautions to students with prior orthopedic complaints. "Such instructions might consist of little more than cautioning the students to avoid activities that produce any discomfort," they said. They added, however, that their findings would not suggest discouraging such students from participation unless they were specifically so advised by their physicians.

TRAINING AND CONDITIONING

Smart aerobic dancers share some of the same strategies employed by safe runners. Adequate warm-up and cool-down periods certainly affect injury rates. Slow and concentrated stretching, without bouncing, should be done for at least five minutes before and after activity; beginners should take ten minutes to stretch. Increasing activity also increases risk; your chance of hurting yourself jumps significantly when you go from three classes a week to four. This doesn't mean you can't add to your weekly regimen, but it does suggest you should do it slowly and carefully. Finally, aerobics are best when they are part of an overall fitness plan. The injury rate of those San Francisco students who counted aerobics as their only fitness activity (39.3 percent) was nearly three times greater than for students involved in multiple fitness activities.

Variety may be the spice of life but it is the main entrée of physical fitness. Although one of the strengths of a well-designed aerobics class is that it will exercise all the major muscle groups, this is also one of this activity's weaknesses. If you have certain muscle deficiencies, an aerobic dance routine is not concentrated enough to focus on this personal weakness. Aerobic dance improves tendon elasticity, muscle efficiency, vital capacity, and resting heart rate. It can also decrease the percentage of body fat, lower blood pressure, improve body cholesterol, increase scalp hair density (Really!), improve range of motion, and enhance one's general sense of wellbeing. That is tremendous, but it can't do everything! What it may not do is make specific muscles strong enough to prevent injury, although it certainly can create injury.

For example, aerobic dance will provide some hamstring and quadriceps strengthening, but if you happen to have a special deficiency in one of these muscle groups—caused perhaps by an earlier injury—you may not be able to focus enough time and energy in a general class to bring those muscles up to their protective best. Many aerobics students prove this themselves when they try another workout, say bicycling, swimming, or running, and then face surprisingly sore muscles.

Individuals who participate in several activities are likely to be better conditioned and more limber, more attuned to their bodies' strengths and weaknesses, and better able to withstand the negative stresses that go along with any sporting activity than their friends and associates who focus on just one activity. They also have shown a commitment to fitness. Which means that as good as an aerobic dance program can be for you, there's more to fitness than showing up for class three times a week.

SHOES

An image that makes any professional shudder is a young instructor in tights leading a barefoot aerobics class on a cement floor. The best foundation for your efforts is a wooden floor laid over several pads of cushioning. But be careful: A wooden floor over concrete is just as bad as concrete alone.

You not only have to wear shoes, you have to wear the right shoes. You can get by with tennis shoes if you have to, but running shoes are no substitute for aerobic shoes. When you're running your shoes are designed to grab the running surface, providing stability and forward control. Such a shoe can be a real hazard to the anatomy if used for aerobic dance. An aerobics shoe needs to provide cushioning and some control, but running shoes anchor the foot too much for aerobics, especially the side-to-side movements so popular with the latest "soft" aerobics. (See Chapter 17.)

The biggest reason aerobic dance is such a pain in the knee is that its movements are exactly the opposite of what you and I were built for. In walking and running you land on your heels, rock forward to the balls of your feet, and then come off of your toes. That's what your body was designed to do. However, in aerobic dance there's a complete reversal of this normal motion. Rarely do you move forward. Instead you're always fighting your momentum and landing on a spot that's not meant to take such force, namely, the balls of your feet. Which is another reason why you do *not* want to wear running shoes: Runners need extra cushioning at the heel rather than the ball of the foot.

PREVENTING INJURY

What was true for runners in the last chapter is equally appropriate for aerobic dancers: The vast majority of injuries are avoidable. The major failings of aerobics fans includes inadequate warm-ups and cool-downs, plus unflagging efforts to push harder and harder in order to "go for the burn."

Not surprisingly, the number one problem is overexercise. In the San Francisco study 80 percent of the complaints were injuries of gradual onset or overuse. There is a physiological point of diminishing returns. For the average person twenty to thirty minutes of aerobic activity three to five times a week is recommended. Beyond this the cardiovascular benefits are minimal, but the number of orthopedic injuries rises exponentially. Indeed, most aerobics-related injuries occur after twenty-five minutes of continuous activity. (To better understand the physiology of injury, see Chapter 19.)

COMMON AEROBIC INJURIES

Here's a look at the most common aerobic dance injuries.

Chondromalacia Patella

At first it occurs as slight annoying kneecap pain within hours of activity. Soon it occurs during activity and the dull aching pain may eventually sideline you if left untreated. The knee bends of aerobic dance are the best at provoking symptoms. Prolonged sitting will also cause stiffness and aggravate your condition. If you happen to have feet that pronate or tend to roll toward the inside, you are at greater risk of chondromalacia patella. (For more details, see Chapter 5.)

If you have chondromalacia, there is a softening of the underside of your kneecap and the nerve endings there start complaining. For treatment, rest from aerobic dance is essential. Although symptoms may be cyclic, with periods of no symptoms followed by flare-ups, once chondromalacia has set in you will need to take some corrective measures.

Part of the problem is that your thigh muscles (quadriceps) are weak, injured, or just out of balance. This disrupts the normal smooth action of the kneecap and causes the irritation of it. Exercises that improve quads strength will also improve patellar tracking and reduce pain. Anti-inflammatory medication, such as aspirin, warm soaks, and elastic sleeve braces worn during activity may also be helpful.

Patellar Tendinitis

This condition is also known as "jumper's knee," which explains why aerobic dance participants are susceptible. You're at much greater risk for this disorder if you train on a very hard floor.

A pain, at times sharp, around the kneecap is usually exacerbated by jumping. There may also be swelling, redness, and warmth around the patella. To differentiate this from chondromalacia, try straight-leg raises. These should be quite painful if you have patellar tendinitis but not so if your problem is chondromalacia.

Aspirin, ice/friction massage, and avoidance of pain-causing activity are the primary methods of conservative management. (See Chapter 5.) Shoe orthotics may also be beneficial for some people. A program of prevention should include adequate warm-ups, stretching of the quadriceps and hamstring muscles, ice packs after especially vigorous training sessions, and careful choice of training and surfaces. This latter means a surface with some "give" to it. Suspended hardwood floors are the safest dance surface, providing maximum shock absorption with a minimum of foot instability.

SOFT AEROBICS

Within the last couple of years another option has emerged for individuals worried about the injury rate of regular aerobic dance. Instructors have seen the lite. Now the buzz words are "noncompressive," "controlled," "soft," "low-impact," "nonimpact," or "lite" aerobics. Here, side-to-side marching, dance-walk combinations, or gliding movements are substituted for the jolting up-and-down motion of typical aerobic routines. Music still sets the pace, but the tempo is likely to be slower. And light weights, as well as giant rubber bands, are often incorporated into the workout.

In soft aerobics one foot stays in contact with the floor at all times, which eliminates much of the jarring impact associated with traditional routines. Movement is kept lower to the ground, with the body's pressure against the floor creating isometric resistance and conditioning. This approach strengthens muscles, develops elastic flexibility, and increases stamina without stressing the joints. There is also an increased amount of armwork, mostly above the heart, which can increase cardiovascular loading by 20 percent without undue stress placed on bones and muscles. The mere act of bending your knees, for example, lowers the risk of injuring muscles and tendons, and that same bend in your routine also works the hamstrings in the back of your leg, which is one muscle group that is too often neglected.

But Are Soft Aerobics Safer?

Glowing testimonials aside (which, after all, are sponsored by the people who want your money), instructors often design low-impact exercises that are not natural to the way people normally move, which means this form of exercise could lead to a new set of injuries. For example, overzealous arm flailing could cause hyperextension injuries to your shoulder. If you already have knee problems, even the reduced weight-bearing exercise of low-impact steps could be intolerable. Since this approach involves putting all your weight on one leg or the other at all times, chondromalacia may still be a threat. And because movements are often exaggerated, a lot of stress is placed on the knee, ankle, and lower back, meaning problems in any of these areas will likely be complicated by soft aerobics.

Are Soft Aerobics as Effective?

A study presented at the American College of Sports Medicine meeting in 1986 indicated that while high-impact exercise gives a more intense—and more beneficial—workout, low-impact aerobics meet the minimum criteria for quantity and quality of exercise as described by the association of sports medicine specialists. Still the biggest health problem associated with this movement may be related to the health benefits you'll lose if you don't pay attention. You're increasing your heart rate, mostly through isometric tension. If you go through the motions in a mindless fashion, your heart rate won't go up and you'll lose the aerobic conditioning benefits of the activity. Concentrating on the task at hand also allows for rhythmic, continuous motion without forced effort. There's even an added plus: maintaining conscious control over movement—even when tired—helps keep your joints in a safe range of motion.

Some instructors encourage the use of hand-held or wrist weights to increase workout intensity for already fit students, although ankle weights are not advised. If you are prone to stress fractures or knee problems, overloading with ankle weights will make it worse. In fact, the side-to-side movements associated with soft aerobics significantly increase the torque (twisting) that goes into the feet and legs, which means ankle weights could increase the risk of knee injury.

Soft aerobics are so new that there's little data available on injury risks. Some instructors claim you can work out longer—forty minutes or more—with greater safety and less stress on the body. Still, the injuries to avoid are overuse injuries, and since soft aerobics can provide the same aerobic conditioning as regular aerobics, there's no point in courting trauma by lengthening your routine.

The American College of Obstetrics and Gynecology recently issued guidelines for the average exerciser. They suggest that heart rate not exceed 75 percent of the recommended maximum; classes should be no more frequent than every other day; the aerobics portion should be limited to thirty minutes; and no more than four hops should be performed in sequence on the same foot.

Some students worry about the soft reputation of low-impact aerobics. They fear that they're not getting the workout they feel they need. If that's the case, perhaps the ideal regimen would be a weekly combination of both styles of exercise. And if you are looking to increase your activity level, perhaps the safest route would be to add on low-impact aerobics rather than going for any more burn. That way, you probably won't *be* burned.

Whichever aerobics style you choose, remember that your risk of injury is reduced considerably if you simply exercise a little common sense.

KNEE SAVERS

- If you have a knee problem, bent-knee activities such as squats or kneeling on the floor are inadvisable.

- Don't do aerobics barefoot, period. Also, use an aerobics shoe and not a running shoe.

- When initiating an aerobics program, limit your workouts to 30 to 45 minutes, no more than every other day.

- Find a class that is suited to your level of performance. Don't fight to keep up with the class leaders.

- Plan enough time for proper stretching before your workout. If you miss the warm-up, do not jump right in! Take some time and prepare your muscles for activity.

21

Skiing:
The Glide Guide

Recently while examining the woes of the weekend jock, a sports medicine clinic at Saint Francis Memorial Hospital, San Francisco, found that the knee was the site of the most injuries and that weekend skiers had the most knee problems. In fact, skiing causes more injuries in general than any other sport, including football. More overall injuries are seen among Alpine or downhill skiers than cross-country skiers. Later, however, we'll explain why cross-country may actually be the biggest hazard to knees.

Several aspects of the skiing experience have undergone considerable change in recent years, but there's still room for improvement. For example, while modern technology has made ski bindings more reliable, many injuries still result from improperly adjusted or maintained bindings. Another problem is the social climate of the sport—skiers often hit the slopes after hitting the bottle, which tends to make a hazardous situation a potentially disastrous one. But even cold sober, skiers often jeopardize their skiing trip, and especially their knees, by not exercising—among other things—caution.

ALPINE OR DOWNHILL SKIING

Downhill skiing is popular around the world: There are 14 million skiers in North America alone, another 10 million in Japan, and an even greater number in Europe. The lines at the ski-injury clinics are also pretty staggering: 250,000 skiers are injured annually in the United States. As painful as that figure is, that's a major improvement from the seventies, when there was a 41 percent decrease in the overall ski injury rate between 1972 and 1978. The improvement is a result of many factors, including innovative advances in equipment, more widespread ski instruction, and better ski-area management.

Interestingly, as the incidence of ski injury changes, the pattern of injury is also changing. The good news is that of all injuries, those to the lower extremities have been reduced most dramatically. The bad news is that serious knee injuries have increased significantly. During the last couple of decades, one type of lower leg injury, the spiral tibial fracture, has been reduced in frequency by 79 percent and ankle injuries are down 82 percent. Yet, at the same time, the knee remains perplexingly vulnerable, with ski injuries to the knee consistently ranging from 20 to 35 percent of total injuries, depending on whose study you're reading. That's bad enough news for knees on the slopes, but it gets worse. A five-year investigation of Vermont skiers, for example, indicates that 28 percent of all injuries now involve some damage to the anterior cruciate ligament compared to only 5 percent in earlier studies. So with tibial fractures and ankle injuries both diminished by almost 80 percent, knee ligamentous injuries are now the most common ski injury. (In case you're wondering, fractures of the thumb are in second place.)

Why? Ironically, one reason knees are still at considerable risk is that the improvements that save thousands of fractured legs and sprained ankles each season could be putting the knee in greater jeopardy. In particular, boots today are built higher and with less flexibility to provide greater control of the ski and more protection for the ankle and tibia. Unfortunately, solving one problem has created another: The torque, or twisting, that once would have injured the ankle or lower leg is now being transferred up the leg to the knee. The resulting injury isn't even comparable to a simple fracture. Bone will mend and the individual will regain most if not all of his or her original strength in that limb. But a ruptured knee ligament will not heal on its own and will require extensive rehabilitation to even approach its former ability to support its owner.

If you'd like to avoid all this, the research says that you probably can. The major causes of injury are exhaustion, poor conditioning, and poor technique. But before these are addressed, we must start at the beginning—with you.

Body Check

If you're physically fit, skiing is less strenuous and more enjoyable, your performance will improve faster, and you'll reduce your risk of injury. Generally speaking, few conditions are contraindictions to skiing. Many people in their seventies still take great pleasure in hitting the slopes. Of course if you're a skier over fifty, regular physical exams are recommended; if you're new at skiing and over forty, you should also get a checkup. And if you have a history of heart or lung problems, or chronic illness such as diabetes or vascular disease, you, too, had better see your doctor before heading for the hills.

If you tend to be loose-jointed, you should probably concentrate on developing strength to avoid sprains. If you're tight-jointed, you should devote extra time to stretching and flexibility training to reduce your chance of suffering a painful muscle pull.

Minor variations in your foot posture can make a major difference in your skiing technique, and thus affect your risk of injury. Small degrees of imbalance become significant when they affect the skier's posture and ability to turn. This is fairly common, according to data compiled by Steven Subotnick, a doctor of podiatry and a professor of biomechanics and surgery at the California College of Podiatric Medicine. He reported in *The Physician and Sportsmedicine* (10:1, 61+, 1982) that 80 percent of thirty skiers he studied failed to have proper edge control due to various biomechanical abnormalities of the lower extremity. Another study of more than 1,000 skiers also found that four out of five rode their outside edges excessively.

Orthotics can be used inside downhill ski boots to aid in parallel skiing. Cants can also be of value to skiers. A cant is a wedge of plastic that fits between the bottom of the boot and the ski. The bindings are mounted over the cant and adjusted to allow for safe release tension. Cants can help skiers who have problems initiating turns and holding on to a hill of ice.

As is true in many sports, some of the problems facing skiers have less to do with inherent difficulties than they do with poor choices made during outfitting. As Dr. Subotnick noted, beginning and recreational skiers of average or below average ability tend to buy unnecessarily expensive and stiff ski boots that accentuate the forward lean and may cause pressure problems for the less skilled skier.

Even the best-outfitted skier is a disaster waiting to happen unless he or she is properly conditioned. Unfortunately too many skiers are too inactive for most of the year. Suddenly the season appears abruptly with the first snowfall and they're calling on their muscles to perform feats that they simply aren't prepared to manage. This can put a damper—if not a cast—on a skiing trip. You, however, can be an exception to the rule. Here's how:

Conditioning

First, before hitting the slopes, remember that they can hit back with a vengeance. While skiing might appear to be a less than demanding sport—after all, it is all downhill, right?—in reality it is one of the most demanding sports.

Before you send your knees downhill, you should work on your endurance, your strength, and your flexibility. Endurance training is necessary to prepare for sustained periods of activity, skiing included. Remember, exhaustion is a key factor in injury. Strength training is also very important, especially for the quadriceps and hamstrings, which protect the knees and legs. Your natural skiing position—with bent knees—is an unnatural position that makes demands on leg muscles that are simply unprepared for the challenge. Moderate abdominal strength is necessary for proper balance control, and upper extremity strength is required for pole action, balance, and maneuvering. And flexibility training will protect you against muscle strains, which can occur when your legs suddenly shoot out from under you and you do "the splits."

Jogging and rope jumping are excellent for endurance training. Knee extension exercises with progressive ankle weights develop strength in the quadriceps. (See Appendix A for more ideas.) Using your ankle weights as you flex your knees from a standing position up toward your buttocks is helpful for developing hamstring strength. (There is one important proviso to using ankle weights: If you are prone to knee problems or stress fractures, the use of ankle weights is not advisable. If you strap ten pounds on your ankle and carry it from ninety degrees [which is your flat-footed position of sitting] to full extension, you are transferring 920 pounds across your patella. This is a great way to unwittingly detect chondromalacia—the screams give it away every time. So use ankle weights only if you're the owner of two healthy knees.) The bent-knee sit-up is good for strengthening the abdominal muscles. See Appendix A for appropriate stretching exercises, too.

Conditioning implies starting out slowly and building up gradually. The amount of conditioning you'll require depends largely on your overall physical shape. This doesn't mean that you have to be an athlete in order to safely put on skis, but it does mean that if your idea of aerobic activity is a quick run to the refrigerator during commercials, maybe you better just stay home and watch the *Wide World of Sports*.

Technique

While we can't give you instructions on these pages, we offer you two hearty words of advice: "Take lessons!" Finding a good instructor is gliding in the right direction. You need to understand the basic ups and downs of skiing: how to fall and how to get back up again. You also need to know the fundamental techniques of skiing, the special equipment that will provide you with the safest trip (literally as well as figuratively), and advice on your form or lack thereof. A lesson each trip will refresh you and maybe even save you from some serious pain.

Bindings

Today's downhill ski bindings are a huge improvement over the cable bindings of twenty-five years ago, but their safety is dependent on proper selection, installation, adjustment, and maintenance. Ideally, bindings lock your boot to your skis until the moment of a fall, when you must instantly break away to prevent injury. Of course premature binding release can be just as dangerous as no release at all. As hazardous as skiing is, it's even more treacherous without skis. To avoid accidental release, most modern bindings use a two-mode release system that provides classic toe rotational release as well as forward twisting release. Older systems had forward lean release, but the newer bindings include rotation at the heel, which is a primary factor in protecting your knees. Such protection is available in multidirectional release bindings, but fewer than 20 percent of the skiing population use this multimode release system. The standard practice is to encourage only beginners to use such bindings, which will release with up to six different force applications. However, that may be severely limiting the best available protection.

Of course it would also be nice if the bindings that were being used were used and set correctly. Studies indicate that too many skiers are skating on pretty thin ice when it comes to the safest setting for their bindings: All levels of skiers studied are at potential risk of injury because their bindings are set higher than recommended.

That's especially true for advanced skiers. It's common for skiers who think they are improving rapidly to decide on their own to adjust their bindings from a five to a seven. This drives the skiing industry (and their insurers) nuts! Skiing retailers spend thousands of dollars and countless hours in special industry classes learning how to set bindings. Skiers who adjust their own bindings truly risk life and limb. They are told this at every turn, but when an accident occurs, they sue the people who sold them their equipment, the people running the ski area, the person who planted the tree that jumped out in front of them, everybody they can think of except the one party responsible for the accident: themselves.

If you think your bindings need adjusting, ask an expert. If you just got your skis and there's premature release, take them back to the shop where you bought them. Many shops will make an adjustment like this free of charge.

The release problem for beginning and intermediate skiers is likely to be related to the condition of the bindings. It's a real temptation for skiers to run a couple of hills and then take a break for a trip to the lodge. While making the trek to and fro they clomp around getting their boots caked with mud, then they climb back into their bindings. What they don't realize is that contaminated bindings can increase what's called the "din" setting, or release setting, by two. Thus, your bindings may be properly set at five, but if you get the whole system buried in mud you effectively have a din setting of seven, which means you'll be in real trouble when your bindings don't release on time.

Similarly, skiers who are using old gear that hasn't been calibrated recently could also be a couple of din settings off. In fact, if you have an old bindings system that is numbered only one through four, and you haven't had them calibrated recently, those numbers probably mean absolutely nothing. The springs in bindings lose their strength over time and bindings set eight years ago at a din of four may now only have a din of two. So I would say that half of the beginning and intermediate skiers I've seen are using either outdated bindings that need recalibrating (or, better yet, replacement) or they're sailing around in filthy bindings that are not going to respond favorably in a spill. It is estimated that 40 percent of all lower extremity injuries in skiing result from the failure of the binding to release properly.

If you have already suffered a ligamentous sprain, you should, as a precautionary measure, have your bindings set so they can release more quickly than normal. That's because once you've been injured, it will take much less force to do much more damage. This is especially important for the two to three ski seasons immediately following the injury. And if your knee isn't fully recovered, an appropriate protective brace may be in order.

If you are in the market for bindings, here are some guidelines you should follow:

1. Choose a binding that has a release adjustment that corresponds to your weight. Your required release setting should be just above midrange on the bindings indicator scale.

2. If your bindings are new, have their release setting adjusted by an authorized technician.

3. Purchase bindings that release in as many modes as practical, regardless of the type of load encountered.

4. Check for compatibility. There are a number of components to release-retention systems, and while they may be purchased separately, not all of the components are structurally or functionally compatible. For example, a toe from one binding and a heel from another can be like having radial tires on the front of your car and regular tires on the rear.

5. You should be outfitted according to your height, weight, athletic ability, and snow conditions. More important, tell the clerk what kind of skiing you do. There are three types of skiers, generally recognized by three letters: L, A, or S. The letters really don't stand for anything anymore, but they do still distinguish three different types of skier.

The "L" skier tends to ski slowly and is always under control. Once the letter stood for someone just learning how to ski, but many skiers who have been hitting the hills for ten years or more still use this particular approach.

An "A" skier was once thought of as "advanced," but all it really means is that the skier enjoys a style that is more varied and aggressive, and terrain that's probably more difficult than an L prefers, but an A skier still remains in control.

The final type was once considered a "senior" skier, but I prefer to think of the "S" as standing for "speed." These individuals don't ski as much as they *attack* a hill. Their control is generally all in their minds. Unfortunately it's their bodies that get spread out all over the runs when they have a blow-out at sixty miles an hour.

6. If you don't know the difference between a din setting and a table setting, be careful where you shop. While specialty stores generally employ well-trained personnel, chain-store clerks may know little about skiing. Ask whoever is helping you how often they ski. If they're not skiers, ask to see somebody who is.

7. To be assured that your bindings are of the best quality and are properly mounted, maintained, and adjusted, you must educate yourself about product quality. The best way to do this is by reading articles and maintaining a strong relationship with a really good ski shop. And again, *don't adjust your own bindings.*

8. Keep your bindings clean and lubricated and check them routinely to make sure all safety features are working properly. Every twenty skiing days a skier should check his bindings and lubricate them with a silicone binding spray.

9. You can be price conscious because the cost of most bindings is based on convenience and cosmetic features. However, avoid buying the cheapest bindings because they can lack many important safety features. Also, don't buy last year's models. Each year improvements are made and you want the best protection you can get.

A Bit on Boots

Boot selection is as important as binding selection, for modern boot styling has contributed significantly to the reduction of skiing injuries. The boot should be comfortable and fit properly. Like a running shoe, an improper fit can cause blisters and increase the risk of injury. There should be minimal movement of the foot within the boot and the boot should distribute the load on the leg both in forward and backward leaning. Also, as noted earlier, make sure your boots match your skiing ability.

COMMON SKIING INJURIES

The two most common knee injuries are both sprains: one is to the medial collateral ligament (MCL) and the other the anterior cruciate ligament (ACL). Back in Chapter 6, when we discussed the official American Medical Association categorization of sprains, we mentioned that there were three grades of sprains. The most common knee injury in skiing—and, according to some authorities, the most common injury in skiing—is the mild sprain in which you suffer microscopic injury to the ligament but it is still intact. The moderate sprains are the next most common. In this type of injury the ligament has been pulled so hard that it has actually lengthened enough to produce mild instability. The most severe—and least common—sprains actually feature a partial or complete ligamentous tear. (A common mechanism for this Grade 3 injury is catching a ski tip in deep snow and falling sideward. The skier feels or hears a pop in the knee and is sure that something devastating has happened, possibly a fracture. However, after a few minutes he or she typically stands, shakes the leg, decides that it is not injured that badly, and continues down the hill. Not until the skier arrives at the bottom, or perhaps even after a second run, does the knee begin to hurt and swell.)

Falls in general are a common cause of ski-related knee injury. During a fall many different twisting mechanisms contribute to injury. That's one reason it is not always possible to get a reliable explanation of just what happened from the skier. Of course even if the skier can go into painful detail, it's still difficult to diagnose a tear of the anterior cruciate ligament.

Most isolated ACL ruptures can be treated without surgery. In fact, most recreational skiers can get along quite well without an ACL because skiing is done in a slightly bent knee position, so there is little chance of subluxation (partial dislocation). The main problem associated with missing the ACL diagnosis is further injury. When an ACL sprain is not recognized the skier is not properly rehabilitated and fully 25 to 50 percent of the injured leg's muscular strength may be lost. So an ACL decifiency can place additional damaging stress on other knee structures such as the menisci. Such a dynamic duo of injury almost always predisposes an individual to osteoarthritis. If a rehab program is followed, an ACL injury can be managed and the recreational athlete can be returned to near normal skiing capabilities. (Unfortunately this does not include truly competitive skiers, who have been known to take an early retirement following complete ACL disruption.)

There are a few other knee injuries associated with skiing, including other sprains, meniscal tears, and patella fractures, but these probably account for less than 20 percent of the injuries to the skiing knee. Fortunately, like every other activity we've talked about, almost all of these injuries could be avoided with proper conditioning, proper gear, and avoidance of fatigue.

NORDIC OR CROSS-COUNTRY SKIING

In the early eighties many active Americans decided that this country had been going downhill long enough. The time had come for cross-country skiing. Physiologists call cross-country skiing the most perfect form of cardiovascular exercise. It offers smooth, fluid, total body motion, which exercises upper as well as lower muscles and seems to allow higher heart rates to be obtained more easily than jogging or cycling. Subsequently, a cross-country skier may burn 600 to 1,000 calories an hour, depending on their size and activity level. (Downhill skiers burn, on average, 400 calories an hour.)

Nordic skiing is cheaper, easier, better exercise, and a more intimate social experience. (It is, after all, easier to catch someone's attention when he's not bulleting down a long run and easier to hold someone's attention when she's not in line with a hundred other shivering skiers.) Brochures heralding the wonders of the cross-country experience all trumpet the same cliché: If you can walk, you can cross-country ski. Wear and tear on joints, tendons, and ligaments is actually quite low, making it appropriate for people with arthritis or physical handicaps. It is also a sport that is particularly suited for family and lifetime participation. Another factor affecting the growing popularity of cross-country is the belief that you're much less likely to land in a hospital emergency room, no matter how high your klutz factor. However, despite the relative ease of learning, there are risks inherent with even cross-country skiing.

In cross-country or ski touring only nonrelease-type bindings are used and this can make for awkward conditions when it's bottoms-up. After a couple of dozen spills during the first hour of activity, and contortions that send friends into fits of hysterics, many beginners wonder, "If you can walk, why ski?" Falls during cross-country skiing are certainly less traumatic than most alpine dives, since there's no speed to speak of. The actual time spent sprawled on the earth is dependent on coordination, conditioning, and the particular path you've chosen.

Preparing to Cross-Country

If you want to work on coordination, rope jumping is a good exercise. Bench jumps help develop power, balance, and agility; each helps protect your knee (and the rest of you!) from injury. Start with a small object, such as a phone book, and jump rapidly from side to side across it until fatigue develops. You can gradually increase the height of the obstacle up to about a foot.

As with downhill skiing, conditioning includes endurance activities such as running or aerobics, knee extension exercises with progressive ankle weights to develop strength in the quadriceps, and simple quadriceps setting exercises that you can do by alternately tightening and relaxing your muscles while seated at a desk or watching television. Toe raises, which are especially good for your calf muscles, are very helpful for the cross-country skier. If weights are used, both calves may be exercised simultaneously. If weights are not available, putting the entire body weight on one foot at a time will help obtain maximum benefit from this exercise. (If any exercise causes pain, back off and stop doing the exercise at that level.)

Another good exercise is to lie on your side, your back, and your stomach (not all at once, obviously) and do leg lifts for your lateral thighs and hip extensors.

The path you choose is also important. Most downhill runs are kept well groomed and many cross-country trails can also boast of good maintenance records, but the fact is, there are still endless obstacles appearing when you least expect them whenever you are skiing. And since most cross-country skiing is just that, trekking over hill and dale as opposed to an actual trail, one's trip can be just full of surprises. So while the trees aren't coming at you at forty-five miles per hour, there are other hazards that make cross-country skiing a heads-up sport. But don't worry, if you're not looking for road hazards, they'll certainly find you.

CROSS-COUNTRY INJURIES

Few studies have examined the injury rates for cross-country, but one Swedish study offered an interesting conclusion: Cross-country may actually be more hazardous to knees than downhill. By evaluating 420 ski injuries, the authors reported that cross-country and long-distance skiing actually produced more knee injuries (24.7 percent) than downhill (11.4 percent). I have to add that this was not a large study and thus the figures could be misleading. I certainly see a lot more downhill patients than cross-country, but then there are perhaps five times as many alpine skiers. What else could explain the results? The cross-country crowd tended to be a little older, which could contribute to the injury rate. Fatigue could also influence the figures. Cross-country looks deceptively easy, but in fact it requires more energy than any other popular activity.

SCARED OF SKIING?

Whichever means you choose to go slip slidin' away is up to you, but don't let all this talk about the hazards of skiing keep you indoors all winter. While both types engender some risk, the Consumer Product Safety Commission, which ranks equipment-related injuries, actually gives skiing a pretty good bill of health. They place it about fiftieth on their list of hazardous activities. (Bicycling breaks away as the biggest risk to life and limb.) Put another way, injury rates at the best downhill slopes stand at about 3 per 1,000 skier days. For perspective, consider that ice hockey has an injury rate of 24 per 1,000 in the pee-wee leagues and 250 per 1,000 in professional players. The incidence of reported injuries in children in or around school are 17 per 1,000 and college football has a 1-to-1 injury rate. So while there is an element of risk, don't let that scare the skis right off of you.

KNEESAVERS

- Be sure that you have been outfitted by a knowledgeable source.

- Clean boots and bindings carefully, then keep them clean.

- Fatigue is a factor in most ski injuries. If you're tired, sit this run out.

- This is a heads-up sport. Cross-country skiing especially seems deceptively safe. Keep an eye out for obstacles in your path.

- Do not mix booze and snow, or the next one on the rocks could be you.

22
Basketball

The subject of knee injuries in sports often conjures up an image of a fleet-footed running back whose fleet gets clobbered by a 250-pound tackle. Well, once college and high school fields are left behind, there are two misleading elements to that image: the sport and the participant.

After graduation, aching basketball knees become one of the principle woes of the weekend jock. In a comprehensive 1985 study of 10,000 recreational athletes treated at the Center for Sports Medicine at Saint Francis Memorial Hospital, San Francisco, 46 percent more basketball injuries were seen than football injuries. Furthermore, the incidence of injury by age was reversed: 64 percent of the football injuries occurred to participants under twenty-five years of age, while 62 percent of the basketball injuries occurred to individuals over twenty-five.

In professional basketball the ankle is still the number one injury site (18.2 percent of all injuries), with the knee a close second (14 percent), but guess what causes the most missed games? In one seven-year review of pro basketball injuries reported in the *American Journal of Sports Medicine* (10:2, 16–18, 1982), ankle injuries caused only 18 percent of the games missed, while knee injuries were responsible for a whopping 66 percent of games missed.

The recreational basketballer's injuries tend to differ significantly from pro pains. The ankle comes in a poor second to the knee in the injury department. In fact, knee injuries to the recreational basketball player are greater than the next four injury sites combined (ankle, foot, leg, and spine).

Body Check

Age seems to influence the incidence, and to a degree the severity, of basketball injuries. In the young, injury is often compounded by incomplete growth. Many youngsters have the size of players several years older but often their joints and musculature are not nearly as advanced and, indeed, may even be a little behind their own age group. And, at the other end of the spectrum, old injuries often return to haunt players old enough to see their own youngsters on the court. Sometimes it's not so much the original injury itself that causes a problem but the lack of appropriate rehabilitation. Residual muscle weakness has been documented for years after an injury, which means millions of once-injured knees are today at serious risk of reinjury. (See Chapter 14.)

If you're a recreational basketball player, you should be especially protective of your right knee. The statistics indicate that the right knee suffers considerably more injury in basketball than the left. This may be due to more frequent use of the right leg; basketball players often land on their right leg after jumping, shooting, or blocking shots with their right arm. This is also true for cutting and stopping, which appear to be initiated more commonly with the right leg in predominantly right-handed players. What this means is that if you once suffered an injury to your right knee, that same troubled joint is at especially high risk of injury in basketball.

Is this right-leg risk associated with being right-handed? Or to look at the question another way, does being left-handed mean you tend to use the left leg more? Quite frankly, no one has done the studies yet to prove this one way or the other. Part of the problem is that there are too few left-handed players to construct a significant study. Logically, it makes sense, but realistically we can't say whether being left-handed makes you harder on your left leg in sports. Your best bet would be to pay close attention to your own style or have someone watch you carefully from the sidelines. Do you tend to lead with one leg more than the other? Do you land on one leg more than the other? If you do, you had better make sure that it's not your "weak" leg or you are just asking for trouble.

Conditioning

Your best bet is to make sure that your legs are both peak performers. Do a muscle check and see if you need to work on your legs. Go to Appendix A and do a series of straight-leg raises, starting with the leg that you consider to be your best. Do as many leg raises as you can. Then repeat with your other leg. Is one considerably stronger than the other? If you're out of balance, work on strengthening both of them. You may find after a few weeks of straight-leg raises that your "good" leg could be even better, which means more protection against injury, especially for your knee.

As long as you're active and supplementing your basketball with other activities, such as running, walking, biking, aerobic dance, etc., you won't have to maintain your straight-leg raises indefinitely. Most people find that after about six weeks they are fine-tuned enough to maintain their stronger muscles by means of their regular activities. If, however, you are rebuilding following major muscle loss associated with an injury, you may have to work on your legs for three months or so before they are back in shape.

And whatever you do, don't rely on basketball, or any other individual sport, to fill all your fitness needs. Maintain a conditioning program or your next bank shot could mean an early withdrawal from the game.

COMMON BASKETBALL INJURIES

A number of factors seem to be involved in basketball injuries: (1) jarring repetitive movements—running, jumping, sudden stops and starts—on unyielding playing surfaces; (2) intensive conditioning and training techniques; (3) prolonged competitive periods or longer seasons; (4) protracted athletic careers, especially for professional athletes; (5) a tendency to continue these activities into adulthood for physical fitness and recreation; and (6) skeletal malalignments of the lower extremities.

The incidence of injury has little to do with the position played. According to a report in the *American Journal of Sports Medicine* (10:1, 16–18, 1982), no one position is safer from injury than any other. However, the *type* of injury is influenced by position. For example, guards suffered more lower extremity injuries, with knee injuries in particular making up almost half of their injuries over the seven years studied. Forwards suffered mostly upper extremity injuries, such as to the head, fingers, and hips. Centers were treated to a combination of upper and lower extremity injuries, with the knee coming in second for attention behind the head.

Patellar Tendinitis

The most common basketball knee injury is "jumper's knee," or patellar tendinitis, which we discussed in Chapter 5. For a long time physicians believed that patellar tendinitis was a self-limiting adolescent affliction that did not cause significant functional disability. Guess again. In a review of 300 cases (in which I participated), we found that this condition will not necessarily go away on its own and it's not always easy to treat.

There are progressive stages to this disorder: (1) It begins with pain only after activity. At this point there really is no functional disability. (2) Then pain begins to be experienced both during and after activity, but still there's little functional disability. (3) Finally, the pain does interrupt one's game and eventually sidelines the player. (4) If the condition is left to deteriorate further, the final phase leads to nonstop pain, on or off the court, and a possible "catastrophic" rupture of the involved tendon.

If caught early enough (while still in phase one or two), jumper's knee responds well to reduced activity, ice massage after activity, heat on the knee at night, elastic support, judicious knee exercises, and a short course of aspirin. Occasionally, if the problem persists, a single localized injection of a steroid may be used. However, once you have trouble walking or running and suffer pain both before and after activity, then a "career crisis" may occur in the pro and a "recreational crisis" may affect the amateur. The alternatives are generally surgery or giving up the activity.

Sprains

Torn ligaments, or sprains, are also common in basketball. Women are especially susceptible, with one Canadian study (*International Journal of Sports Medicine*, 6:314–16, 1985) showing that women suffered five times more ruptures of the anterior cruciate ligament than men. (In this study ACL injury accounted for one fourth of all basketball injuries in women.) Again, greater emphasis on women's strengthening programs could shrink the injury rate for women considerably.

Sprains often occur in basketball when you land on another player. Sprains are ranked in three grades (1 to 3): mild, moderate, and severe. The pain is localized in the first two sprains and diffuse in the more severe third. Meniscal injury is also fairly common along with a sprain. The best treatment is immobilization (with crutches or a brace), ice or cold packs, and a rehabilitation program.

Patellofemoral Pain

The kneecap often complains when it's attached to a basketball player. The problem is generally either chondromalacia or a subluxation/dislocation condition. These conditions share many of the same symptoms. The most distinguishing feature of the latter problem is a feeling that the knee is going to collapse. In either case strengthening the musculature of the leg can help relieve symptoms and allow a return to pain-free action.

Finally, there is one contributing factor to basketball injury that seems to affect kids of all ages. There's this interesting human trait that tends to ignore injury. We "tough it out," "be a sport," "don't let a little pain bother us." When our kids do it we call it "immaturity." When we do it we call it "taking care of ourselves." Remember what they say about people who act as their own attorney in court? There's also no fool like an old fool—especially one blithely ignoring pain or injury.

KNEESAVERS

- Precede *every* game *and* any break of fifteen minutes or more with a good stretching regimen.

- Check playing surfaces for uneven areas or wet spots.

- Wear basketball shoes with good support and plenty of cushioning. If your shoes are worn out, get a new pair fast.

- This is an anaerobic sport, so players are often in oxygen depletion. Proper condition is crucial.

- Remember, fatigue often leads to injury, and basketball is a grueling and fatiguing sport.

- Players should get proper fluid replacement while playing.

- No wide loads! This is not a good sport for the overweight. The combination of excess pounds and intense bursts of activity places a great burden on your knees, your heart, and your general metabolism.

23
Tackling the Problems of Football

Before we look at the good news, here are the statistics: Approximately 1 million high school students play football and each season approximately 40 percent are injured. According to one review of sports injuries reported in the *American Journal of Sports Medicine* (14:3, 220+, 1986), football is the most common sport of injury with greater than twelve times the number of injuries seen in the next most common sport, basketball. The Occupational Safety and Health Administration puts it this way: A football player—either high school, college, or pro—is 200 times more likely to be injured than a coal miner. The majority are not serious injuries, although one in four does require more than a week off the field for recovery. Most studies suggest that the knee is the most common site of football injury (up to 42 percent) and all studies concur that it is the leading injury requiring surgery and the most common cause of permanent disability. Each year there are up to 130,000 knee injuries among professional, collegiate, scholastic, and sandlot football players, and 30,000 to 50,000 require surgery.

Football and Arthritis

For a long time there has been a common assumption that competitive sports activity is linked with early osteoarthritis. We've already pointed out that statistical analysis has found this to be an overstatement. Professional soccer players and even veteran military parachutists have all been carefully studied and, despite torturous activity, these individuals show no greater incidence of osteoarthritis than the general public. Now we can add football to the list of strenuous and bruising activities that do not automatically lead to pain, degenerative changes, or disability to knees decades after leaving the playing field.

If a football player does, however, incur a knee injury, there is a rather ominous prognosis: Eventual disability is very likely. The North Carolina researchers who looked at both the soccer players and parachutists (*British Journal of Rheumatology*, 25:243–52, 1986) found that nearly half of the football players who had suffered a knee injury during their high school days showed radiographic (X ray) changes suggesting the development of osteoarthritis. There were no differences in the functional capacity of any of these young men compared to uninjured controls—at least not yet. According to the investigators, "Based on the history and radiographs, one would be concerned that over the next ten to twenty years, a significant disability might develop."

OFFSIDE AND HOLDING AN INJURED KNEE

For a long time many doctors didn't really care about soft-tissue injuries, such as ligament tears, because they weren't life- or limb-threatening. But in later life these injured athletes were finding themselves faced with stiff and painful joints that were causing major quality-of-life problems. The real tragedy for these aging athletes is that so much could have been done to avoid their deteriorating condition.

Today correctly diagnosing a knee injury is considered one of the most important challenges facing sports medicine. Unfortunately it's not as easy as it might seem. If a player is writhing on the ground in pain and grabbing his knee, it doesn't take a Harvard Medical School graduate to tell you something may be wrong there. The real challenge comes when the player gets up, hobbles around for a few minutes, and then declares that he's all right. If the injury happens during a game, there's generally a physician to double-check the young athlete's self-diagnosis, but if it happens during a practice session, there may be no medical authority to run interference on behalf of an overly eager youngster. And here we run smack into a major problem: Most grid injuries occur in practice.

In February of 1987 the National Athletic Trainers' Association, Inc. (NATA) released the results of perhaps the biggest prep sports-injury survey they've ever conducted. They collected data from 105 schools participating in the National High School Injury Registry and then projected nationwide figures based on the 6,544 high school players in those schools. Their results: Injuries sidelined 37 percent of the nation's 1 million high school football players at least once in 1986 and 62 percent of those injuries occurred during practice.

INJURY PREVENTION

The NATA is convinced that one way to stem the incidence of injuries is to have more athletic trainers serving our young athletes. Athletic trainers are not doctors, but often they do have training in the proper conditioning of athletes and attending to their pulls and strains. "We would never even consider putting a professional club on the field for a practice or a game without a trainer," said Dr. Allen Levy, the New York Giants' team physician and a guest of the NATA during the announcement of their study. "But we do it all the time with our children. It's my feeling that our kids bleed just like the pros do."

Of course athletic trainers aren't the only answer. Jerry Rhea, president of the NATA, feels that four factors contribute to the high number of time-loss injuries in high school sports: disparity in the size of the athletes, lack of experience, lack of knowledge about conditioning, and poor-fitting or overused equipment.

BETTER CONDITION MEANS FEWER INJURIES

In 1978 researchers reported that a closely supervised, high-quality, preseason conditioning program resulted in a significant reduction in the incidence and severity of high school football knee injuries (*American Journal of Sports Medicine* 6:180–84, 1978). A later study (*Illinois Medical Journal*, 166:5, 356–58, 1984) found that preseason conditioning slashed the number of athletes requiring hospitalization for conservative treatment of knee injuries by about 75 percent and reduced the incidence of early season knee injuries by 67 percent. Conditioning also meant fewer days lost following injury for most athletes.

Too many of the schools that do incorporate preseason conditioning into their football programs abandon them at the beginning of the season in favor of drills and scrimmages. Yet we know that conditioning, particularly flexibility, is lost without continued effort. Furthermore, conditioning doesn't just happen in a few preseason weeks. Athletes who do not begin to stretch until the beginning of a season will receive minimal benefits, if any, that season. It takes time for flexibility to develop, but when it does it offers considerable protection against injury. Thus, conditioning should be a year-round goal for the young athlete.

An even more immediate goal is to get players through a game with proper warm-up. Before the game there's no problem. The team gets out on the field and takes great pride in spending ten to fifteen minutes showing off their stretches, exercises, and warm-up activities. During halftime, though, they go into the locker rooms and sit in cramped conditions listening to the coach's pep talk. During this time they are losing much of the flexibility they developed during the initial warm-up and first half of play. Then they run back out on the field, perform a couple of perfunctory stretches, and jump back into the fray. I suspect that many of the injuries that occur during the third quarter could be prevented, or at least they would be less severe in nature, if there was as much of an emphasis on warming up before the second half as there is prior to the game.

Is the game safer than it was a generation ago? Yes and no. I think it's safer as far as rules, equipment, conditioning, warm-up periods, amount of time players are on the field, and expertise of the coaching staff. However, the players are bigger, faster, tougher, meaner, and they try to emulate the pros. One of the basic equations of physics is "mass $\times$ acceleration = force," and today the forces in high school football are much greater. So if it were not for definite safety improvements, our young athletes today would really be facing a war zone out on the football field.

New regulations have been especially helpful in increasing player safety. Seven rule changes were specifically designed to reduce knee injuries. Among them, rules against blocking below the waist, chop blocking below the knee, running into the kicker, crackback blocks, and changes in the legal clip zone have all managed to contribute to a safer game for all players. These rule changes, however, require proper officiating to see that the players abide by the rules.

THE KNEE INJURIES OF FOOTBALL

But, no matter what, some injuries will occur. Internal derangement of the knee is the leading football injury. You may recall that I.D.K., as it's called, means that something (or several somethings) inside the knee have been torn, crushed, stretched, or otherwise injured. This catchall category is followed in frequency by patello-femoral injuries, sprains and strains, fractures, and inflammatory conditions. Any football player sustaining a knee injury that is disabling—even for a moment—should be suspected of having incurred a major ligamentous injury in the knee. This becomes almost a certainty if the player recalls being hit with the foot planted and the knee slightly flexed. Once the diagnosis is made of a complete ligamentous tear of the knee, surgical intervention with repair should be carried out within the first ten days. After this period of time, repair is more difficult and less sure.

Once the injury has been recognized promptly, treated by repair or reconstruction, and the athlete has been rehabilitated, normal athletic activity is often possible, although no reconstruction will have the complete power and control of the original equipment.

The immaturity of growth plates in youngsters makes them uniquely susceptible to two medical problems: Osgood-Schlatter's disease and epiphyseal injury.

The former is also known as "football knee." It's more likely to strike the junior varsity player and is associated with repetitive stresses inflicted upon still-developing cartilage plates. The pain is most often found at the front end of the tibia, just below the kneecap. Running and jumping aggravates this condition. Fortunately it responds well to limited activity, quadriceps strengthening exercises, and cold applications. (For more on Osgood-Schlatter's disease, see Chapter 26.)

The growth plate, or epiphysis, is a weak link in younger knees. As we age and stop growing, this plate fuses with the bone. Then if a force tears into the knee, it will be the ligaments that are first injured, not the bone. For youngsters, the situation is just reversed: Their ligaments are five times as strong as their growth plates. The turning point for boys is about fourteen years. Thus, it's the youngest pigskin players who are at greater risk of epiphyseal injury.

About 10 percent of all childhood skeletal trauma involves an epiphyseal injury. Fortunately, if diagnosed properly and managed well, these injuries do not lead to uneven growth. That is a risk, however, so an epiphyseal injury must be taken seriously. (For more information, see Chapter 26.)

This look at football underscores several of the problems facing high school athletics in general. It only begins to hint at some of the problems of all scholastic sports. In Chapter 27 we'll take a quick look at some specific problem areas and what can be done to save young knees.

24

A Six-Pack of Sports

Tennis elbow may be the most famous, but now there are more sports-specific pains than there are sports. Some of the best known include: jogger's toe, cyclist's palsy, footballer's ankle, jumper's knee, billiard player's finger, bowler's thumb, racquetball player's pissiform (a personal favorite in the name game), musher's knee (from kicking behind dog teams), and hooker's elbow (we're talking ice fishing here). Certain sports and activities present particular hazards to participant knees. Here's a look at the knee hazards lurking behind several popular pastimes.

BICYCLING

Although Detroit has spent much of the last decade backpedaling since new-car sales hit the skids in the late seventies, another vehicle's business has been wheeling right along. Bicycles have become the recreational vehicle of the eighties. With bike sales exceeding car sales in recent years, it's estimated that one of every two Americans now owns a two-wheeler.

If your bicyclist image is a teenager with a paper route, think again: Today the average member of Bikecentennial, the nation's leading two-wheel tour organization, is thirty-five years old, with a median family income of $30,000.

That's the good news. We now must face the fact that the bicycle is the most common cause of product-related death and injury in the United States. According to the Consumer Product Safety Commission, cycling is the most dangerous athletic activity in America. Each year there are nearly 450,000 hospital-treated injuries involving bikes, compared with only 400,000 in baseball and football. Nearly 20 percent of these accidents are caused by mechanical failure, generally because bikers don't take care of their machines. However, according to some authorities, improperly sized wheels or frames and poorly adjusted seats or handlebars may cause more accidents than mechanical failures. Even if you don't have an accident, you can accidentally injure yourself. Although many people with knee problems turn to bicycles for recovery workouts, cycling is not as benevolent to your knees as you might think—especially if you're a woman.

Body Check

Knee pain is the most common complaint among bicyclists. Knock-knees, bowlegs, or pronated feet put additional stresses on the knee. Therefore, bicyclists with even slight degrees of these anatomical variations can injure ligaments or bursas and aggravate chondromalacia patella, one of the most common problems associated with bicycling.

If your toes naturally point in or out instead of straight ahead, you have a greater risk of patellar tendinitis. Forcing your toes into an unnatural (for you) straight-ahead position mile after mile may strain the kneecap's most important tendon. If you think your body could cause you this type of problem, you might want to see if orthotics could help you prevent injury.

Likewise, individuals with knock-knees may build up the inner sides of their pedals or shoes and/or use arch supports to relieve some of the strain on the medial collateral ligaments or mild chondromalacia. Similarly, those with bowlegs may obtain relief of pain in the lateral collateral ligaments by building up the lateral (outer) sides of their pedals or shoes.

Women may be more susceptible to the knee effects of two-wheeled workouts. Their wider hips mean that their thigh bones connect to their hips at a wider angle than men, which means they don't line up as directly over the shins and feet, and that causes added stress on the knee joint with each pedal stroke.

Fitting Yourself to a Bicycle

To explain bike fitting, I use my underwear analogy. Without thinking, many people borrow a ten-year-old's ten-speed, ride around for an hour, and get off complaining how uncomfortable the darn thing is. Yet these same people would never borrow a youngster's Fruit of the Looms, wear them a while, and then declare Fruit of the Looms just too uncomfortable.

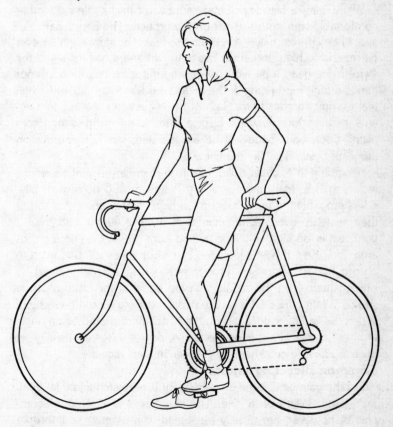

Women may find it more difficult to find the right bike if they insist on a drop frame (the old "girl's bike"), which has a smaller selection of sizes. But unless you're planning on wearing a skirt when you ride, you're probably better off buying an appropriately fitted diamond-frame bike (the old "boy's bike"). Besides offering a wider choice of frames, a well-fitted diamond-frame bike actually provides the better ride. Drop-frame bikes, without that top tube, are often too springy and less durable. In any event, visit a good bicycle shop and also ask about other bikes that many women are finding to be the perfect fit, such as mixte frames (top bar is attached at an angle) or all-terrain bikes.

When fitting a bicycle first make sure you can straddle the top bar comfortably with both feet flat on the ground. The handlebar stem should be approximately level with the seat. The stem should never be raised too high. If there is less than two and a half inches of the stem in the head tube, you risk having the stem break off in your hands during hard riding. If the measure is less than two and a half inches, buy another stem. Both of these elements are key ingredients to fitting yourself with a bicycle. If the fit is improper, the forces acting upon your body will be exaggerated, which is murder on innocent bystanders like the knee.

According to Michael Kolin, coach to many top American riders, including U.S. team member Cary Peterson, "90 percent of bike riders probably put their seats up too high" and women tend to put their seats up even higher than men. What's wrong with this? If your seat is too high, you'll be putting extra pressure on your crotch area. However, if your seat is too low, your knees will be forced to absorb the extra stresses. Proper saddle height is determined by sitting squarely on the saddle with the pedal at the bottom of the stroke. When your heel is on the pedal, your leg should be straight. When the ball of your foot is on the pedal there should be an angle to your knee of about fifteen to twenty degrees. (Racers usually set their saddle one centimeter to two centimeters higher.)

Common Bicycling Injuries

For the younger set the most frequent bike-related injury is "road rash" from falling off a bike. The older, recreational riders' complaints, however, are usually associated with overuse or improper fit. Overuse is a particular hazard today. Driven by an interest in fitness, many people turn to bicycles for an enjoyable aerobic workout. Unfortunately the "no pain, no gain" mentality has made cycling murder on the knees.

With knee pain leading the pack of bikers' complaints, it should come as no surprise to find chondromalacia patellae, patellar tendinitis, sprains, strains, and bursitis the most common injuries among riders. The patellofemoral joint, which is where the patella and the femur (thighbone) come together, is under particular stress. Much disability could be prevented if the early, often subtle, symptoms of knee distress were given prompt attention. Most important, riders need to gear down when their knees hurt.

A classic case was a man who lifted weights as a youngster to gain muscle bulk. Using the same philosophy later in life when he started biking, he made it a point to use the large gears, pushing hard to gain strength in the legs. He may have had the strongest legs in town, but he almost ruined his right knee.

If you do suffer from chondromalacia, you may have to stop riding and do everything possible to prevent excessive pressure between your kneecap and thighbone. Training on flat terrain during recovery is also important, as is maintaining proper cadence and applying ice after training. Besides correcting the cause of the problem, such as improper fitting of the bicycle, remember—if your knees hurt—gear down.

Bursitis is often confused with chondromalacia. The bursas are tough membrane sacs that fill with fluid and flair up under irritation or injury to cushion friction points throughout the body. By pushing too hard on the pedals, bursas can be injured, causing painful swelling. The synovial membrane surrounding the knee may also become irritated and cause swelling, with or without bursa abuse. (For more details about these medical conditions, please see Chapter 5.)

Your particular riding form will also affect your knees. When viewed from the front of the bike, your knees must be pointed forward, not inclined toward the top tube. The latter is not at all uncommon, particularly among competitive riders. Wind resistance is the greatest force the racer has to overcome, and in an effort to become more streamlined, the rider will bring the knees inward toward the top tube. The predictable consequence is knee pain.

Spring is also hard on the knees, or at least the way many bikers

ride into the season. After months of weight lifting or other alternative activities, bicyclists often resume training or trailing where they
left off in the fall. If you want to keep your knees happy, take it easy
and reenter spring training slowly.

Getting into gear is not that difficult. With a little knowledge and
some preventive medicine, bicycles can remain a thing of beauty
and a toy forever.

KNEESAVERS

- Make sure your bike is fitted to your body.

- Beginners should stay on flat surfaces and use comfortable gear
  settings.

- High gears are a bad workout for your knees. If your knees
  hurt, immediately gear down and check your riding posture.

- If you've got chondromalacia patella, avoid high gears, hills,
  and toe clips.

WRESTLING

Although television has given wrestling the image of a live-action
cartoon, injuries associated with wrestling are not funny. Wrestling
consistently shows a significantly high injury rate, often second only
to football. In virtually all reports, injuries to the knee account for a
sizable proportion of total wrestling injuries. The range has been
from 5 to 27 percent. Several studies have found it to be the
number one injury site.

But whether the knee was the most frequently injured site or not,
when a wrestler suffered a knee injury, it tended to be more serious
than most other injuries. In perhaps the most detailed study of knee
injuries associated with wrestling, a six-year review of injuries sustained by the University of Iowa wrestling team found that the
average number of days lost per knee injury was 18.8 days. This
contrasts sharply with nonknee injuries, which, on average, cost the
player only 6.8 days.

During the six years of the study the Iowa team was the NCAA champion five times. Knee injuries comprised 27 percent of all injuries sustained over the period. One reason for the high rate of knee injuries might be the fact that more emphasis is placed on takedowns at the University of Iowa, which makes it more akin to freestyle wrestling than the mat wrestling approach of most other teams. Takedowns appeared to put the knee at greater risk of injury, and defensive wrestlers appeared to be at greater risk during the takedown. The wrestler "underneath" was also injured more often.

Common Wrestling Injuries

Sprains and strains are the number one pain among wrestlers. This suggests a need for improved flexibility training, which can be beneficial in preventing such injuries. Conditioning for strength, as well as power, can also be instrumental in preventing joint injury. And training for muscle endurance should be emphasized. Matches may not take long by the clock, compared to other activities, but the intensity of the action can tire muscles quickly.

Strains and sprains often occurred during takedowns, which makes sense since there is an increased vulnerability at this point and there is much more practice time spent doing takedowns. The lead leg, which is the leg closest to the opponent, didn't appear to be at any more risk than the trailing leg, at least not during takedowns. That's in sharp contrast to meniscal injuries, which were almost exclusively found in the leg that the wrestler generally used as his lead.

Meniscal injuries were also distinctly different from many other sports. Several of the meniscal injuries appeared to be more degenerative tears than traumatic. The authors of the study, which appeared in the *American Journal of Sports Medicine* (14:1, 55–66, 1986), hypothesized that the "knees of these young wrestlers undergo in a short time stresses that occur in nonwrestlers over a much longer time period." Wrestling, in effect, rushes the biologic clock and the accumulation of "microtears" quickly leads to injury.

Overall, the authors reported that the lead leg *is* at greatest risk of injury because of the greater stresses it faces, however the trailing leg, when injured, generally is hurt more severely because the wrestler is less able to counter his opponent when that back leg is attacked.

Perhaps the most frequent wrestling injury is prepatellar bursitis.

The bursa on the face of the knee is injured by either a single traumatic event (a knee slam into the floor) or repeated trauma. Treatment for the pain, swelling, and tenderness includes rest, immobilization, padding, draining (aspiration), and compressive dressing. Unfortunately, once afflicted, a wrestler may find the problem recurring. Eventually surgery may be necessary to remove the irritated bursa.

According to data from the University of Iowa, prepatellar bursitis appears to be more common in the lighter weight classes. As a group the lighter weights spend more time "shooting" at their opponents' legs (forget the artillery, this has to do with going down on one or both knees while attacking the opponent) compared to the upper weights, who use throws and moves not involving knee contact with the mat.

Conditioning and Rehabilitation

The knee is most at risk during matches, which have forty times the injury rate of practice, with matches early in the season being particularly risky. This suggests that proper conditioning, especially during the off season, can be protective against injury. Proper rehabilitation once an injury occurs may also be another means of preventing injury. The Iowa team showed that wrestlers with previous knee injuries were twice as susceptible to a second injury. Unfortunately rehabilitation is often not a priority for young wrestlers. The research showed that when the Iowa wrestlers were injured they didn't often listen to their doctors' advice and their noncompliance rate was nearly 50 percent, considerably higher than that found in most other sports. Was there a price to pay for this? Indeed. Those who didn't take their rehabilitation seriously were more than twice as likely to get injured again. It's ironic, because when athletes enter a rehabilitation program, they do beautifully, but when they return to action too soon or ignore their doctors' medical advice, they can pay an awful price in pain and further injury.

Is this college data equally applicable to high school and recreational wrestling programs? In a commentary accompanying the published study, Dr. Joseph Estwanik of Charlotte, North Carolina, believes that most of the data is probably applicable to other programs. However, the facts and figures need to be kept in perspective. As the authors point out, catastrophic knee injury, such as a tear of the anterior cruciate ligament, was low, and the severity of injury not as great as that found in football.

Preventing Injury

Since this study offered new insights into the specifics of knee injury in wrestling, this will lead to further investigations and perhaps more specific preventive measures that will eventually make the sport safer. Until then the keys to injury prevention include: (1) a good conditioning program, especially off season; (2) better supervision of rehabilitation efforts; (3) an emphasis on mat wrestling as opposed to freestyle wrestling; (4) improved conditioning, endurance, and (especially) flexibility training.

KNEESAVERS

- Most injuries occur with fatigue. Call it quite before your body does.

- Use foam knee pads to protect from mat abrasion.

- Maintain your flexibility with appropriate stretching between matches. A good warm-up, followed by lengthy periods of inactivity, is not sufficient.

GOLF

Many golfers have a two-handicap: their knees. Although for some people nothing can be more relaxing than eighteen holes, you don't generate a club-head speed of 100 miles per hour in less than a fifth of a second while falling asleep on the links. A variety of acute and chronic problems can dog anyone on the course, and many of them seem to nip right at the knee.

Body Check

Eleven million golfers now play fifteen rounds or more a year in the United States, and along with the graying of the nation there will probably be more golfers queuing up for tee-off times. While team sports participants are often young, healthy, and in good condition, golfers come in all shapes, sizes, and ages. Yet golf is a throwing sport, even if you don't send your clubs sailing into a water hazard. Golf includes the torque and countertorque of the discuss thrower, the reflex thrust of the javelin thrower, and the joint stretch and body rotations of the baseball pitcher. Just thinking of all of that may make some people sore.

Any golfer with a weak knee, a weak back, or any other weak area is at greater risk of golf injury and should focus strengthening programs on these areas. Fatigue also adversely influences coordination and reflexes, thus contributing to injury. Limit your golf swing to what your tissues will bear.

Part of the problem is related to the evolution of the golf swing. In *The Physician and Sportsmedicine* (September 1976, 42–47) three golf authorities explained, "The older or classic golf style of the Jones-Hagen era in the 1920s was characterized by a long flowing backswing, a large hip turn, and a collapse of the left wrist at the top using whippy, hickory-shafted clubs.

"The finish of the swing was a relaxed straight up and down or 'I finish,' which achieved a competitive end result with less physical strain. Since that time, leading professionals have made technique changes with modern equipment to gain greater distance with more accuracy. But these techniques are physically more demanding and less suitable for the average player of today."

Common Golfing Injuries

That means today's hard-driving man and woman can face a number of physical problems. Perhaps the biggest is that acute golf injuries are judged minor when compared to other sports injuries and therefore they tend to receive less attention and inconsistent medical care. Subsequently, such inadequately treated injuries can create chronic conditions that are extremely difficult to correct.

While imagining your own golf swing, here are the most common complaints: bursitis (associated with forces created during both preimpact, impact, and postimpact), patella instability (due to preimpact forces), and synovitis (inflammation of the synovium caused by postimpact forces). Fractures are uncommon in golf, but one case history offers an insight into the forces of the golf swing and the special hazards of this sport, particularly to the once-injured athlete.

Following a college basketball injury, a young man underwent a reconstruction of his anterior cruciate ligament. Six months postoperative, he had good range of motion, showed no signs of instability, and wore a Lenox Hill brace for activities. At this point his activities were increased slightly to include hitting golf balls on a practice range, primarily with short irons that don't require much knee rotation. No problem—until he decided to try a couple of shots with his driver. On his very first shot he felt a pop in his knee, followed by pain and swelling. X rays showed a transverse fracture of the patella. Ouch!

Preventing Injury

Sometimes these problems will be best relieved by making corrections in your form. If your stance is unnatural, for example, the forces going across your knee may be several times what they should be. Occasionally these complaints are actually caused by unrehabilitated (and sometimes unrecognized) old injuries. However, perhaps the biggest problem is the classic sporting deficiency: poor conditioning. Walking is good exercise, but specific exercises to enhance both quadriceps and hamstring strength could go a long way toward preventing some of the aches and pains associated with playing golf.

Strains occur when the muscles are not fluidly flexible as a result of either insufficient warm-up or cold-weather contraction. These are also common among golfers. Prevention means proper warm-up, a series of stretching exercises, and exercises that emphasize strength and flexibility. While sheer strength alone won't enable a player to hit the ball better or longer, it will allow a skilled player to strike shots with more consistent explosive power over more extended periods.

The easy pace and apparent limited physical action and exertion of golf are deceiving. Although many people take up golf because they are in "poor physical condition," as in any sport, the injury rate is tied to the condition of the players. Don't make golf an excuse to keep from getting into shape. Handicap your game, not yourself.

KNEESAVERS

- Get in the groove. Warm up with chip shots and drives that will facilitate your eye/brain/muscle coordination.

- Check your footwear. Make sure your spikes are clean and none are missing.

- Watch where you're walking! One of the worst knee injuries I've ever seen was inflicted on a golfer who stepped into a hole.

SWIMMING

Swimming, both recreational and competitive, remains the most popular participatory sport in the United States in the 1980s. Although swimming produces fewer acute accidental injuries than contact sports such as soccer or basketball, the risk of overuse injuries may actually be greater. Such injuries, you may recall, are due to repeated stress caused by excessive motion or impact shock. The result is microscopic damage, which, over time, becomes more and more significant until finally symptoms appear.

The competitive swimmer is at risk partly because of the incredible training sessions that are required for the sport. Many top swimmers now swim 12,000 to 20,000 meters per day (approximately seven to twelve miles). However, it is not necessarily the distance traveled nor the time spent in the water that actually put the athlete at risk, but rather the mechanics and the intensity of the swimming that initiate the problem.

The breaststroke is the oldest competitive stroke and one of the oldest swimming styles. Much of the speed achieved in the breaststroke comes from the kick, so particular emphasis is placed on the development of an efficient and powerful kick. Of all the kicks swimmers can use, the whip kick has been shown to be superior in every respect, including speed and propulsion force. It is also the kick most commonly taught to breaststrokers at all levels of competition. Unfortunately, if done incorrectly, this technique can cause "breaststroker's knee."

Common Swimming Injuries

Breaststroker's knee refers to a sharp pain, generally localized to the inner aspect of the knee. Initially symptoms are restricted to whip-kick activity. However, as the swimmer continues to use (or misuse) the breaststroke despite discomfort, the knees become painful during other athletic and nonathletic activity. Discomfort has specifically been linked to stair climbing and activity requiring squatting or heavy lifting with the knees bent.

Although most often seen in the young, competitive swimmer, elite swimmers are not immune: studies have shown that even when the proper technique is used, the severity and number of repetitions alone can cause knee problems. Poor technique, however, is probably the biggest cause of this complaint.

Treatment for "Breaststroker's Knee"

This is an inflammatory condition caused by irritation of knee ligaments and can usually be best treated by analyzing the whip kick and making any necessary corrections in technique. That, however, is easier said than done, as often both coaches and swimmers are unaware that the kick is being done wrong.

Rest, ice, anti-inflammatory medication, and strengthening and stretching of the muscles in and around the knee may also be helpful. During recovery it's important that other kicks be substituted for the whip kick during workouts, although in advanced cases of breaststroker's knee most kicks will cause some discomfort.

If not promptly and vigorously treated, a number of researchers have warned that swimmers may suffer serious and disabling knee problems. For example, breaststrokers who have been using poor form for a number of years show clinical evidence of patellofemoral osteoarthritis. Chondromalacia patella (which by now should be an old friend of everyone reading this book) is also a risk for whip-kicking swimmers.

Although a wide variety of operative procedures have been performed on swimmers with breaststroker's knee, none are even remotely as successful as merely correcting faulty technique.

Preventing Injury

Sometimes the problem is that the athlete is actually doing an illegal breaststroke kick, almost a scissor kick with the legs unequal in the water. But generally the kick is not illegal, just poorly executed. Fortunately, if caught early enough, the swimmer can be retrained and his or her knees can be saved further abuse.

Besides correcting technique, proper warm-up may also prevent breaststroker's knee. A minimum of 1,000 to 1,500 yards of warm-up has been suggested before hard breaststroke training begins. Increase in breaststroke training distance must also be gradual to prevent acute knee pain. Alternating other strokes with the whip kick during training programs is also recommended. And, particularly for the elite competitive swimmer, two months of total rest from swimming is suggested during each year.

WEIGHT LIFTING

Most men in the United States, along with a growing number of women, have at some point been involved in some form of weight training or weight lifting. A typical student's use of weights is as a supplemental program to improve performance in another sport. Once school is out, grown-ups who hated P.E. have no qualms about shelling out several hundred dollars a year for health-club memberships, which generally include access to Universal or Nautilus machines. Although a dedicated athlete can use such circuit weight training for strength improvement and perhaps some cardiovascular benefit, most people use this elaborate equipment for more of a general or overall workout. Finally, weights can be used for body conditioning. This is the individual who pumps a little iron now and then to "stay in shape," but hasn't really had any formal instruction in weight lifting. These people comprise the majority of weight lifters. (There are, of course, many competitive weight lifters, such as body builders, Olympic weight lifters, and power lifters who are often highly trained athletes using weights as a means to their own end.)

The noncompetitive weight lifter typically uses lighter weights and higher repetitions than the competitive lifters and body builders. However, both groups are susceptible to a number of injuries and the knee is a frequent problem area.

One hazardous weight-lifting activity is leg curls. When this exercise is done through a full range of motion, there may be a "click" and a sharp pain near the extremes of motion. Although this particular pain is usually transitory, sports medicine specialists believe this could contribute to future degenerative knee problems such as osteoarthritis. Meniscal tears occur during leg curls, as well as with dead-weight lifting. In one review of forty-three weight training-related injuries, four were meniscal tears and each required surgical repair.

It has been reported that the maximum force across the knee occurs at thirty to forty degrees of flexion, which means that during deep knee bending the force through the patellar tendon is 7.6 times body weight. (Don't bother figuring it out. For a 200 pound man this would mean over 1,500 pounds through a cringing knee-cap.) This is a factor in dead-weight lifting, which requires repetitive knee bends, starting with the knees in a semiflexed position. There is general agreement that knee injuries can result from this exercise and, considering the forces involved, it should come as no surprise that patellofemoral pain is a frequent problem.

Several years ago we got a real clear picture of the forces across the knee during weight lifting when an Olympic contender attempted to clean and jerk a heavy weight and he actually ripped his patellar tendon from the bone. A film was being taken at the time and subsequent analysis showed that at the time of the avulsion the patellar tendon tension was about eighteen times the lifter's total weight.

Body Check

Most bodies, given time, can withstand a good weight-lifting program. However, because of the forces involved, it is especially important that prepubescent youngsters be closely monitored if they participate in weight training. At this age there is no significant increase in strength or muscle mass in boys, probably because there are not enough circulating androgens. However, weight training can, if done judiciously and with supervision, improve speed and agility. The risk is that weight "lifting," which means the lifting of maximal weights, can cause epiphyseal injury, which is injury to the growth plates of developing bones. This is why athletes in Eastern European countries are forbidden to lift maximum weights until the age of eighteen or nineteen. So the concerns for the risks of injury or damage in growing children is realistic.

Common Weight-lifting Injuries

Patellar tendinitis is the most common injury associated with weight lifting. Although this condition is generally associated with jumping, it is more fitting to consider it an overuse problem. Anti-inflammatories, such as aspirin, and ice/friction massage are generally helpful, assuming that the condition is treated in time. Otherwise, surgery may be necessary. Chondromalacia patella is also associated with overtraining. Meniscal tears are a definite hazard for weight lifters, especially during deep squats or in the middle of attempting a clean-and-jerk movement.

By taking weight lifting—or any other activity, for that matter—slow and easy, you'll be much less likely to suffer an injury. If you give your muscles and tendons time to adjust to greater work loads, you should be able to avoid chronic stress-related injuries.

Which Came First? The Weights or the Injury?

The biggest medical problem associated with weight lifting is probably overuse injuries; the biggest challenge for the doctor is determining whether weight lifting caused or merely aggravated an injury. Because the vast majority of weight training-related injuries appear to be injuries of a gradual onset, the athlete will be unable to precisely determine when the problem first appeared. Add in the fact that the athlete is probably vigorously involved in another sport, too, and it's difficult to learn what has caused the problem.

So the researchers from the University of Notre Dame, Methodist Hospital of Indiana, and the Great Plains Sports Medicine Foundation recommended in their journal report that if there is a question as to whether the sport or overtraining caused the problem, the weight-training aspect of the program should be temporarily eliminated while sports involvement continues. If the symptoms disappear, this would seem to incriminate the weight-training program.

Why is this important? Throughout this book we have underscored the insidious nature of many sports medicine injuries. Overuse injuries are so common and have the potential for being so disabling that it is imperative that the development of the problem be understood in order to prevent further injury. From the athlete's perspective there may be nothing more frustrating than an overuse injury. It generally starts quietly and builds, which means in the early stages, when it is most amenable to correction and treatment, it's easiest to simply ignore the problem and hope that it goes away. It is also surprising that even though pain often occurs during the weight exercises themselves, research shows that individuals often do not recognize the association between their pain and their weight workouts until they are specifically questioned about cause and effect.

None of this is to suggest that there is no place for weight lifting in a conditioning or training program. It does need to be understood, however, that the all too common premise that states "if some is good, more is better" is a dangerous one, particularly for young athletes involved in weight lifting. At this point we really don't know what amount of training is necessary to provide optimal athletic performance. Therefore, at any age, anyone involved with weights should be supervised by knowledgeable people who can offer instruction in proper lifting techniques and injury avoidance. Furthermore, it becomes your responsibility to listen when your body talks. If it starts to complain, find out what's causing the problem before it becomes a medical condition that interrupts your activity.

KNEESAVERS

- Deep squats should be limited in frequency, since they are associated with the greatest risk of injury.

- Stretching and flexibility maintenance is vital. Muscle pulls occur when muscles are not supple.

- Post-workout stretching helps clear metabolites from muscles and increases your recovery rate.

- Leg curls are especially hazardous to the knees. Keep this activity to a minimum and don't attempt to overload.

- Weight lifters tend to ignore aerobics, which means ignoring the most important muscle in the body: the heart. Improved cardiac performance will improve your blood's oxygen-carrying capacity, which in turn will improve your weight lifting.

RACKET SPORTS

One hundred years after it was first described in medical literature, epicondylitis lateralis humeri, or tennis elbow, is probably the most familiar sports-associated ailment. Yet a review of over 10,000 injuries presented at a San Francisco sports medicine clinic showed that the leading injury site in tennis was the knee, not the elbow.

Fully 24.4 percent of the tennis injuries were knee-related, compared to 22.2 percent that involved the "upper extremities," which included hand and finger as well as elbow injuries. It's possible that individuals with tennis elbow may have chosen to see their own physicians instead of reporting to the Center for Sports Medicine at St. Francis Memorial Hospital. After all, tennis elbow is not an acute but a chronic condition.

If all other racket sports are considered, then upper extremity injuries probably do lead the pack, with ankles, knees, and shoulders vying for position. But whatever order these injuries are placed in isn't really important. It's obvious that knee involvement in racket sports injuries is significant and worthy of a few minutes of consideration. If you consider the lunging stabs and tortuous pirouettes that are involved in tennis and some other racket sports, it's easy to understand how recreational athletes' knees can be turned into mush on the court.

Body Check

The critical aspect of racket sports is the recognition that all athletics are basically like ballet, which defines the position of the body in space. Without proper form and function, you're at risk of injury and difficulties. A famous illustration of this is how baseball great Dizzy Dean injured his elbow and the injury ended his career. How did he wreck his elbow? Because he broke his big toe. Hang on, it will make sense. His broken toe caused him to change his delivery just enough so that he stressed—and ultimately ruined—his elbow. As a sports medicine physician, I never cease to be amazed at the complex interplay between injuries and anatomical factors. If you look at a slow-motion video of someone hitting a tennis ball, it is balletic. As they are stepping into the ball their weight is transferring, their body is balanced, their left hand is out (assuming they're a right-handed player), and the positioning of the hands and legs, the symmetry and the form and function of the body—it's as beautiful as Baryshnikov leaping onto a stage.

How can the knee affect all of this? In two ways: Either the knee can suffer an injury during play (or due to play) or a knee injury can affect the form and function of play and cause an injury. The latter are your "Dizzy Dean" injuries, that is, injuries that are caused by the "ballet" mechanics of sports. If you have a knee injury or problem, you could be leading off with the wrong leg, you could be striking the ball with your body weight transferred too far forward or backward, and this could cause an injury to shoulders, elbows, back, or hips. I've actually seen tennis elbow that was caused by an unrecognized knee problem. How? He wasn't extending his knee all the way, due to a small meniscal tear irritating the knee. When you favor your knee you may easily find yourself leading off with your back foot or stepping off too soon so that your shoulder goes through the ball before the racket hits it, and eventually you start complaining that your elbow or shoulder hurts.

Preventing Reinjury

In this book we discuss the millions of Americans who are weak in the knees and don't even know it. If you have ever had a knee injury, the odds are that, unless you were specifically rehabilitated, you have one leg that is considerably weaker than the other. That's why you must first rehabilitate your weakened knee and build up your endurance. Then go to a coach to make sure that you are performing the mechanics correctly.

Common Racket Sports Injuries

The most common injuries we see in racket sports are overuse injuries, most often related to playing on hard surfaces and repeated impact with the court. Tendinitis on the medial (inner) side of the knee and bursitis are the two most common overuse injuries.

Tendinitis produces a pain, at times quite sharp, that is exacerbated by jumping. There may also be swelling, redness, and warmth. The first step toward recovery is cutting back the irritating activity, in this case racket sports. Ice/friction massage stimulates circulation and provides some pain relief, as do anti-inflammatory agents such as aspirin. Shoe orthotics, knee wraps, or a "jumper's knee" brace may be beneficial for some people. Stretching and strengthening exercises are appropriate to prevent recurrence.

With bursitis, instead of a tendon becoming enraged, it's one of the bursas protecting the inner side of the knee. If diagnosed early enough, an ice massage after activity may be helpful without having to restrict your activities. However, if left to deteriorate, the condition is best treated with rest for three to six weeks, aspirin, and ice massage. In some particularly difficult cases, some physicians report that a knee splint for four to six days will shorten rehabilitation time. A chronic problem may be alleviated with a neutral orthotic.

What causes these problems? Most likely the fault lies in poor form—for you or your game. We've mentioned a little about your form on the court. Your form in general may put you at risk. If you're overweight, you'll have decreased endurance: Basically your body is spending so much time and energy feeding your fat cells that it can't clear away the waste products from your muscles fast enough to bring in new energy resources. Of course extra pounds also mean extra stress, since the sheer forces driving your body are greater. Think of it this way: It's easier to stop a Volkswagen than it is to stop a Mack truck. Sports safety is a balance of power and weight. Watch your weight and you should have more power and a better-balanced game.

Accidents also occur when players slip on a slick surface, dive into the court or into the wall, or take a wrong step or a never-to-be-forgotten wrong turn.

Another factor affecting knee safety is the surface being played upon. Although slippery surfaces can certainly cause some real damage, ground-breaking research on the biomechanics of tennis have shown that relatively slippery surfaces, such as clay, actually cause *fewer* injuries than high-friction ones, such as asphalt. Apparently, when the foot slips on a slick surface, peak forces generated by sudden stops and turns are dissipated, reducing shock to the body. However, when the surface grabs the foot, those forces get generated right up the leg and a splash of knee pain sends the player to the ground, exercising his or her command of the English language.

Also, a switch from a slow clay surface, which is more common in the East, to a faster court, where the ball comes at the player faster, can throw timing off and again increase the likelihood of injury. Here, too, it's proof that the coordination of the player is just as important as strength and endurance. Unless they're all working together, something can fall apart.

So whether you're a touring pro or a once-a-year racketeer who can't tell a clay court from a clay pigeon, think of your knees before you pick up your racket. Otherwise, your knees may wipe you out before your opponent even has a chance.

KNEESAVERS

- Too many people racing to make their scheduled court time neglect a proper warm-up. It's better, though, to lose five minutes of playing time than five weeks while you recover from injury.

- Warming up on the playing surface will give you a feel for the court and alert you to any hazards, such as slippery spots.

- Likewise, don't jump headlong into killer competition. Give your muscles a chance to get into the game while you bring your hand/eye coordination up to par.

- Keep replenishing your body with liquids during breaks from activity.

25

The Aging Athlete:
Battles of the Weekend Warrior

Reality. What a concept! Although we laughed when a comedian made that line famous, it actually reflects a serious sports medicine concern: As physical realities change, so do the realities of sports. People who have enjoyed sports all of their lives often lose touch with reality as they age. The reality most frequently missed is that your body changes. Even if you're honest enough to admit that you're not the athlete you used to be, you may still push yourself like you once did. The result can be pain and injury.

We're not talking about the sheer ability to participate in and enjoy activity. We *are* staying active longer. However, certain facts about muscle strength, power, and endurance do affect how we respond to strenuous activity, and ignoring these facts heightens the risks facing the recreational athlete.

The reality is that the body starts to deteriorate after about the age of sixteen. At this point we start getting stiffer; our tissues do not have the same elasticity they did in our youth. If you find this hard to take, lie down for a moment and consider that a "mid-sports" crisis can strike as early as age twelve. I remember one twelve-year-old Little League pitcher who came in with bone fragments in his elbow and I had to be the one to break the news to him: He simply couldn't pitch anymore. Sometimes the crisis is injury-based, but at other times it's simply the discovery that one wasn't built for one's dream sport. Such a crisis occurs whenever athletes become aware that they're no longer as capable as they once were or are unable to achieve the goals they've set for themselves. It can happen when you're still in school or it can happen when you're old enough to have your own kids in school.

Aging in general will hamper every athlete in time, yet weekend athletes act as though they are somehow immune to the calendar. Not only are they not immune, they do in fact face a greater risk of forced retirement than the pros. Recreational athletes are injured far more frequently than top athletes—particularly their knees.

Why do knees give out long before aging athletes do? First, people who enjoy athletics are most likely to suffer from overtraining and overuse injuries. These problems can creep up on anyone, from great athletes who depend on sports for their living to weekend athletes. Second, and most important, the problems facing aging athletes are directly related to what kind of shape they're in. Unfortunately, when it comes to an honest assessment of abilities, the worse shape the athletes, the less willing they are to admit there's a problem.

For our own safety we need little reminders that we're getting older, and we certainly have this need filled in spades: agility, flexibility, and speed diminish, stamina and endurance decrease considerably, power and strength need more attention to simply maintain the status quo, and the ''morning after'' becomes a time to forget the day before. Weekend athletes often ignore the warning signals sent out by their bodies: persistent pain in muscles, bones, or joints. Experienced athletes understand that pain is nature's signal that something is wrong and it's a warning to stop. To recreational athletes, pain means they will have to work harder because they're not in shape yet.

The problems are compounded when there is an old injury lurking inside. If an older athlete once suffered a significant knee injury, he or she is probably at five to ten times the normal risk of injury while at play. The problem is not necessarily reinjury. The new injury frequently has less to do with the initial trauma than it does an inappropriate rehabilitation.

If you had a knee injury anytime before 1970 you probably were casted and told to make certain life-style changes—like get out of sports. Rehabilitation was not emphasized.

The result of this is that millions of active Americans are unknowingly at tremendous risk of injury or reinjury. If you were once injured and never rehabilitated, the odds are that you may have as much as a 50 percent muscle deficiency in your once-injured leg. Your legs may look the same, but they are not even close to being comparably protected against injury.

Try this simple test: Sit on a chair and, with your knee flexed, raise your uninjured leg about a foot off the floor. Have someone press down on your leg while you try and maintain the leg's position. You should be able to counter quite a bit of pressure since you're using your quadriceps, the most powerful muscles in the body. Now try the same test with the leg you previously injured. If you can't resist the same pressure as your other leg, you probably have at least a 20 to 25 percent muscle deficiency in that leg.

Now is the time to get into a program of rehabilitation if you fail the test. Even if you do pass, resistance exercises will provide you with more power, endurance, and strength to do activities at a much safer level. This has been proven in every sporting activity that requires physical prowess. You can't simply pick up where you left off when you were a senior in high school. Your muscles aren't the same length, for one thing, and your timing is certainly not the same: You have to rebuild strength and endurance, then comes form and function. Fortunately the better shape you're in, the better your performance will be and the better able you'll be to handle an emergency situation.

If you are an aging athlete, you can, within reason, have it all: the benefits of activity and acceptable risk. Of course this requires an honest assessment of yourself and a dedication to self-protection instead of self-indulgence.

KNEESAVERS

- Don't try to make up for lost time. Twenty years later is *not* the time to try and break your high school sports record or suddenly decide to become a marathon runner.

- If your muscles ache the day after a workout, you tried too much to fast. Don't increase your workout until you no longer ache the next day.

- No pain, no gain = no brain

- Warm up and stretch for at least five minutes before working out. This is especially critical if you work out only once a week.

- If your daily life is largely sedentary and you are over forty, have a general medical evaluation.

PART FOUR
Kids' Knees

26

What's Up, Doc? (Junior Version)

Contrary to what society has come to believe over the last few generations, children are not miniature adults. This is particularly apparent in medicine, where children, for the most part, have completely different needs than adults. In orthopedics, children face a variety of unique problems, mostly associated with their developing musculoskeletal systems.

For example, ligamentous tears are a leading result of uninvited stress in adult knees. However, when a comparable force rips into a child's knee, the weak link is not the ligaments themselves but the growth plate they are attached to. Thus, before a ligament is severely damaged, it will become partially or totally separated from the end of the bone. This is called an epiphyseal fracture, which is named for the cartilage plates located at the ends of long bones. Although the ligaments are saved, the injury needs close medical attention, since a poorly healed growth plate could affect future growth of the leg. This plate hardens with skeletal maturity, thus older adolescents, like adults, will be more prone to injuring one or more ligaments and less likely to damage the growth plate.

The frequency and severity of knee problems in children appear to be increasing. Unfortunately many of the injured youngsters have no easily identifiable problem. Bring up frontal knee pain and it elicits laughter from every orthopedic group. It's nervous laughter. We all have parents bringing children into our offices who complain of knee pain but offer little else to go on. Fortunately most are not true mechanical problems but rather overuse injuries caused by too much activity on still-developing bodies.

Stress syndromes are nearly twice as common as acute injury in adolescent knees. Three fourths of these stress problems cause frontal knee pain, which is also known as patellofemoral syndrome. One factor contributing to this problem is a wholly inadequate stretching and strengthening program for most young athletes, particularly of the quadriceps and iliotibial band. Most adolescent sports do place a lot of stress on the knee, but proper stretching and strengthening would prevent many injuries.

Once an injury has occurred, exercise is often the key to recovery. Sometimes the importance of the exercise program is not stressed enough by the doctor or fully appreciated by the patient. Usually the young people who experience a recurrence of knee pain are the ones who do not continue the exercise program. One method you can use to underscore the importance of exercise involves having your child perform an activity of daily living that causes pain, such as squatting. Then the child stands and holds one or both hands firmly against the front of his thigh as support while squatting. In most cases this markedly diminishes the pain and clearly demonstrates the importance of gaining additional support by strengthening exercises and/or bracing.

Like adults, kids suffer certain typical disorders and conditions. Here are some of the more common ones:

OSGOOD-SCHLATTER'S DISEASE (Also known as "football knee" or "rugby knee")

The Physician and Sports Medicine calls this "the painful puzzler." Although its exact cause is unknown, this disorder seems to be associated with the repetitive stresses of certain sports. Also known as "football knee" or "rugby knee," the condition is most likely to occur between the ages of eight and thirteen in females and ten to fifteen in males. Although boys are affected three times as often as girls, studies suggest this is due to more frequent and more vigorous sports activities and not to gender.

Symptoms

Osgood-Schlatter's disease appears to be associated with the immaturity of cartilage plates, particularly the one at the front end of the tibia. Pain, swelling, and tenderness in this area is generally aggravated by direct trauma, such as a fall or running, kneeling, or climbing.

Treatment

Fortunately this disorder responds well to rest and a restriction of vigorous athletic participation. Exercises to strengthen the quadriceps muscles are also very important. (See Appendix A.) Fewer than one out of every ten young people with this condition will require more aggressive treatment, which includes some type of immobilization until symptoms subside.

Pain medication may actually be contraindicated since no pain may indicate no disease to youngsters, which could encourage a premature return to vigorous activity. Since pain is well managed by limiting activity, this is the best strategy. Occasionally a knee wrap or sleeve may provide extra warmth during the day, while leg elevation in the evening may provide extra comfort.

There's a wide variation in recovery time. It's largely dependent on the severity of the problem at the time of treatment. If a youngster is diagnosed quickly, two to four weeks is not uncommon, but if the disease goes on for some time before medical treatment is initiated, children can take six to twelve months to return to full activity. A few children may be left with a small bump in the area, but in time this generally disappears.

OSGOOD-SCHLATTER'S DISEASE

Common Name	Who Gets It	Where It Hurts
Football knee	Girls: 8 to 13	Just below the kneecap
Rugby knee	Boys: 10 to 15	on the front of the knee

Other Symptoms	What to Do	Often Confused With
Pain, swelling, tenderness	Stop running and jumping	Chondromalacia patella "Jumper's knee"
Aggravated by running and jumping	Cold applications for 5- to 10-minute periods	"Growing pains"
	Quadriceps strengthening	

OSTEOCHONDRITIS DISSECANS

Sometimes a small piece of a big bone starts to die. The area involved may be no larger than a nickel or dime. Such a lesion is believed to be caused by repeated minor trauma, often of such insignificance that the child won't complain. However, if the condition is left untreated, fragments may break off from the lesion and these loose bodies would then float hazardously around the knee.

This entire process is known as osteochondritis dissecans. While this condition can be found in almost any joint at any age, it's most frequently seen in the knees of active youngsters between the ages of six and fourteen. It usually involves the medial femoral condyle, which is the rounded notch at the end of the femur, and sometimes it can affect both knees.

If you think you may have had this problem when you were growing up, pay close attention to your kids. One report (*Orthopaedic Review* X:10, 37–44, 1981), which reviewed four generations of one family, found twelve definite cases of OCD and eight possible cases out of thirty-one members studied. This suggests either an hereditary link or exceedingly bad luck on the part of the study's participants.

Symptoms

The earliest symptom is usually mild, nonspecific knee discomfort with possible swelling following normal athletic activity. Later complaints of giving way, catching, or locking would suggest a separation of one or more fragments. In children OCD generally develops gradually over a period of time. In older youngsters acute onset associated with specific trauma is more common. In this age group, which starts at twelve for girls and fourteen for boys, the initial symptoms are locking, giving way, and swelling.

Treatment

A protective regimen is often all that is necessary. Most youngsters will respond to a few weeks' rest followed by modified activity that does not bring on symptoms. Aspirin and other analgesics are not used routinely, but they may be administered for recalcitrant pain or swelling. The average child remains under treatment for six months. During this time, if restriction of activity fails to control pain, crutches or a removable cast may be temporarily required.

Sometimes arthrography (which is what we call the use of an arthrogram) or arthroscopy or even both may be indicated to assess the integrity of the bone and overlying cartilage.

Most patients under fifteen years old heal if treatment is started before the fragments separate. Once the separation has begun, surgery may be necessary to remove the fragments or they may be held in place with pins, pegs, wire, or screws and then immobilized for six weeks.

Following treatment, 90 percent of patients have a knee suitable for strenuous athletics.

OSTEOCHONDRITIS DISSECANS

Common Name	Who Gets It	Where It Hurts
	12- to 15-year-olds	Usually over the medial or lateral femoral condyle

Other Symptoms	What to Do	Often Confused With
Aching Swelling Locking (later on)	Restrict activity May require surgery	Torn meniscus

PATELLOFEMORAL SYNDROME (Anterior Knee Pain)

Probably the most common knee problem afflicting adolescents is anterior (frontal) knee pain. The cause of this condition is unknown and it is one of the most frustrating problems for patient and physician alike.

Symptoms

Chronic pain in the front of one or both knees is the primary complaint. The pain is often associated with prolonged sitting with the knees flexed, mounting and descending stairs, and vigorous athletic activity. Relief is generally produced by rest and full extension. Upon examination there may be no symptoms at all, except for pain whenever pressure is placed on the patella. Creaking and crunching sounds from within the joint are also a frequent complaint, although there are few, if any, physical findings.

Treatment

Initial treatment for patellofemoral pain usually calls for rest and isometric exercises. An easy conditioning program is initiated next, including bicycle riding, swimming, or light jogging, although the youngsters are told to avoid running, particularly downhill. Many surgical procedures have been proposed to treat anterior knee pain, but there is little evidence that they are more effective than conservative management.

Exercise

This condition is well treated with isometric quadriceps strengthening exercises. In its simplest form this consists of repetitive lifting of the lower limb with the knee in extension. Done several hundred times a day, this simple method is very effective. Relief is usually evident within six to twelve weeks. (See Appendix A for additional methods.)

PATELLOFEMORAL SYNDROME

Common Name	Who Gets It	Where It Hurts
Growing pains	Poorly conditioned athlete	Front of the knee
	Those in squatting sports	
	Girls slightly more than boys	

Other Symptoms	What to Do	Often Confused With
Sensation of swelling	Modify activities	Chondromalacia patella
	Quadriceps exercises	Osgood-Schlatter's disease
		Patellar tendinitis

PATELLA DISLOCATION/SUBLUXATION

The increased incidence of these problems in the younger athlete is mostly attributable to structural abnormalities, such as a slightly smaller than normal patella, or to muscular immaturity.

Often the kneecap will snap back into place spontaneously. The youngster may describe the incident as "My knee went out of joint." For this reason many dislocations are diagnosed as sprains or torn menisci. Further complicating the issue is the classic teaching that patella dislocation is a disorder of females, when in fact it has been shown to occur with essentially the same frequency in males, particularly in the athletic population.

Symptoms

Pain, tenderness, and perhaps swelling along the inner portion of the patella are the leading symptoms. Relief is often given by massaging the front of the knee. The pain is often greatest when the leg is flexed; straightening brings relief. For doctors the key sign indicating a patellar problem is an "acute state of apprehension" noted when an attempt is made to gently move the kneecap laterally. This "apprehension sign," as it's called, means that the youngster looks like he or she is prepared for launch off of the examining table. The *sign* is what the doctor is looking for. Once that look of abject terror crosses the patient's face, the doctor usually does *not* move the kneecap.

After an acute dislocation it is important to determine if a fracture has occurred. Those at greatest risk are the tight-jointed, because it takes more force to dislocate their patellas. Rapid swelling and blood in the knee are both highly suggestive of a fracture.

The key to finding a fracture is often a thorough X-ray examination. Unfortunately the two quick X rays taken in most emergency rooms are poor indicators of patellar damage. You need to see several specific angles, as opposed to general overview shots of the knee, in order to detect a kneecap fracture. So if your doctor suggests more X rays, there's a good reason.

Following an acute dislocation, one out of six individuals will suffer the same problem again, and with each subsequent dislocation it becomes easier and easier for the patella to slip out of its track. Also, after an acute dislocation, one out of three patients will experience an occasional sense of instability while participating in sports.

Treatment

Immobilization is for five to six weeks to allow healing of the stretched and torn fibers around the patella. This is then followed by a graduated program of rehabilitation. The most notable feature of this kind of patellar problem is a wasting of the quadriceps muscles, so returning these muscles to peak condition is a primary goal. (See Appendix A) Then there is a gradual return to activity.

Surgery

If a fracture is confirmed, surgery may be necessary to repair the fracture or remove any fragments caused by the injury. Many specialists now advocate surgery as a primary treatment of acute or recurrent dislocation of the patella, especially if a developmental defect, such as a poorly tracking kneecap, contributed to the injury. I will admit that because of the tremendous force necessary to dislocate the kneecap of a tight-jointed individual, there can be considerable damage caused by an acute dislocation. So for a youngster who is tight-jointed, whose knee is all swollen and filled with blood, yes, then it's probably time to get more aggressive and consider surgery. But as a primary treatment for patellar problems, I think surgical procedures are not recommended.

The patella is really an enigma. Doctors haven't yet found the answer to patellofemoral problems. There are over a hundred operations listed for this in the medical literature; any time there are more than five operations for any given problem, that means that none of them work consistently. Fortunately 85 percent of all patients with chronic patellar instability are amenable to conservative therapy.

PATELLA DISLOCATION/SUBLUXATION

Common Name	Who Gets It	Where It Hurts
Loose knee caps	Ages 14 to 17 Girls slightly more than boys Jumpers	Front of the knee Kneecap

Other Symptoms	What to Do	Often Confused With
Swelling Instability or buckling	Quadriceps exercises Patellar braces may be of benefit Orthotics may help	Meniscal tears Chondromalacia patella

CHONDROMALACIA PATELLA

This is a rare adolescent problem, but a common diagnosis for unexplained knee pain. If there is a definite malalignment of the knee or leg, an acute traumatic blow to the patella, or some other underlying biomechanical abnormality, then chondromalacia patella may in fact be the problem. The use of this diagnosis was best described by Dr. Carl Highgenboten, an assistant clinical professor of orthopedic surgery at the University of Texas, Southwestern Medical School. In *Orthopaedic Review* (X:10, 37+, 1981) he wrote, "A diagnosis of 'chondromalacia patella' often is a diagnosis of wishful thinking and hoping that the patient and his problem will go away or that the patient will adjust or that he will adjust his life so that he will give the appearance of improving."

As a result of this attitude Dr. Highgenboten is convinced that many easily treated causes of knee pain are "not appropriately cared for, dooming the involved patients to pain and/or decreased activity levels. This is not fair to young, active patients, who deserve a thorough evaluation." (For further information on chondromalacia patella, see Chapter 5.)

CHONDROMALACIA PATELLA

Common Name	Who Gets It	Where It Hurts
Growing pains	Unconditioned athletes Runners and jumpers Girls more than boys	Front of the knee

Other Symptoms	What to Do	Often Confused With
Swelling Pseudo-locking Instability	Modify activities Quadriceps exercises Brace may be of benefit	Everything

ACUTE INJURY OF THE EPIPHYSEAL PLATE/LIGAMENTS

When we began our discussion of children's knee problems, we mentioned that children's ligaments are less prone to injury than the developing growth plate they are attached to. These ligaments are not however, immune to injury. At skeletal maturation, which is about twelve years for girls and fourteen years for boys, the growth plate is finishing its maturation and slowly becoming less of an injury factor. Usually, by their mid-teens, adolescents have achieved their full growth and ligamentous injury becomes a threat to their mobility, just as in adults.

Until that time ligaments will often survive an injury intact but the epiphyseal plate will fracture. Approximately 10 percent of all skeletal trauma in childhood involves epiphyseal injuries. Some critics have condemned many childhood and adolescent sports activities because of the possibility of epiphyseal injury and its potential for causing a growth problem. While it is true that epiphyseal injuries will occasionally interrupt growth and lead to uneven growth patterns, this is rare, occurring in 5 percent or fewer of all growth-plate injuries. Still it is important enough for everyone involved in the care of a child to realize that such a disturbance of normal growth is possible and that it may not be identified for months or even years after an injury to a growth center. That's why when your doctor says your child's fracture has healed and normal activity may be resumed, appointments will be made to follow your child's growth at six-month increments for at least two years. This is just good preventive medicine. If a growth problem does occur, the vast majority can be medically managed fairly easily.

Of course epiphyseal injuries do not preclude the possibility of dislocation or sprain. If the forces acting on the knee are strong enough, a ligamentous rupture may occur. Although football gets most of the bad press, ligamentous as well as epiphyseal injuries are also seen in soccer, basketball, skiing, skating, hockey, bicycle injuries, and more. Problems arise when there is a diagnosable problem, such as a sprain, and there is not enough care given to seeking out an epiphyseal fracture, which can be difficult to detect upon regular X-ray examination. That's why physicians are ordering more stress X rays, which are regular X rays but done under physical stress. By gently manipulating the bones, the X ray may reveal otherwise invisible fractures.

A torn ligament is a particular problem, not because it can't be repaired, but because there is an even higher risk of retearing the reconstruction, and once that happens subsequent repair becomes much more difficult. Adults are often more willing to make necessary adjustments to avoid reinjury; they may change to a less hazardous activity or decrease the competitive level at which they are playing. But a particular sport may be very important to a young player and it may be his decision to continue playing. If the young athlete, once aware of the risk, chooses to continue sports participation, leg musculature needs to be kept in top condition and a protective brace may be appropriate during activity.

When an adolescent's ligament has been torn it is treated the same as an adult's. If it is accompanied by an epiphyseal fracture, however, a different approach may be required.

Symptoms

An epiphyseal fracture can be thought of as a deceleration injury. It often occurs with a sudden and severe pain after landing from a jump, as in coming down from a rebound in basketball or following a pole vault, high jump, or broad jump. Pain is fairly constant and not necessarily relieved by rest.

Treatment

Assuming that the growth plate has not been displaced, treatment should focus on rest and protection, and there should be repeated X rays to follow the healing process. Sometimes a brace or cast is appropriate for protection. If the fracture is severe enough and part of the bone plate is beginning to separate, an open surgical procedure may be necessary to fasten down the separation. Fortunately probably 85 percent of patients will be well on their way to healing within three to six weeks. The growth plate is second only to the skin for speed of cell turnover and regeneration, so healing occurs quickly.

ACUTE INJURY		
Common Name	**Who Gets It**	**Where It Hurts**
Fracture	Traumatic injury	Femur or tibia
Other Symptoms	**What to Do**	**Often Confused With**
Marked swelling	See a doctor	Severe bruise
Painful movement		Ligament Sprain
		(epiphyseal injury)

27

Why Are Junior Athletics So Hazardous?

For years sports medicine observers have noted that while sports have not changed, the young athlete certainly has. He—or now, almost as likely, she—is taller and heavier than his father at the same age, capable of running faster and jumping higher and farther.

The change we're most concerned with, though, is the drastic increase in the number of injured young athletes. The sports medicine division at Boston Children's Hospital, for example, reports a tenfold increase in the number of sports-injured patients they've treated during the last ten years. Why? Opinions differ, but there are certainly some clues and, more important, some suggestions about what can be done to lower the injury rates among young athletes.

Today recreational youth sports programs involve well over 25 million children aged six through sixteen. The fact that there are injuries among these sports-minded youngsters is not news. What is news is the fact that we're seeing injuries in nine-year-old girls we once saw only in scholarship-level male athletes. One of the hazards of junior athletic programs is the increased size and weight of today's youngsters. Contrary to popular belief, lightweight athletes do not sustain more serious injuries than their heavier peers. In fact, the heavier, taller, and less agile a player is, the *more* likely he or she is to get hurt. Other reasons why school-age sports, particularly football, are a lot more dangerous than they should be include improper coaching methods, ill-fitting equipment, and a poor understanding of the rudiments of sports medicine and human physiology.

But there are two overriding factors contributing to this growing problem and at first blush they might seem to be mutually exclusive. On the one hand, children are increasingly entering into competitive athletic activities earlier than preceding generations, while on the other hand, kids may be in the worst shape of any preceding generation.

The increased athletic demand on some youngsters goes beyond the traditional contact sports of football, wrestling, soccer, and basketball to such noncontact sports as swimming, gymnastics, track, skating, and ballet. Yet studies consistently show that the health and exercise boom of the last ten years has been a bust as far as kids are concerned. Since the 1970s the level of fitness among America's youth has been drifting downward until the latest figures by the American Athletic Union indicate that two out of three children can't pass basic physical education tests.

A combination of poor diets and passive activities such as watching TV, using computers, and playing video games has lulled youngsters into a state of fitness stupor. After testing 2.3 million students nationwide, Dr. Kenneth Cooper, the founder of the Aerobics Institute in Dallas, reports that one of every four American children are obese. Moreover, kids have shown a significant, documented increase in their percent of body fat and a decrease in endurance fitness since 1975. The latest figures from the President's Council on Physical Fitness finds low levels of performance in key areas of activity such as running, jumping, flexibility, and strength—the very areas of performance that contribute the most protection against sports injury.

So while some youngsters are experiencing greater athletic demand, others are so out of shape that when they do engage in activity they are at a much greater risk of injury. Furthermore, while professional athletes have teams of specialists serving their sports medicine needs, young athletes are largely unprotected. One reason for this hazardous situation is that only recently have we begun to study the overall injury rate for sports activities of school-aged children. Previously most investigators have studied sports-related injuries as they relate to equipment, selected sports like football, boxing, or baseball, and the "older" school athletes. One of the biggest failings of such studies has been the total lack of insight into pre-high school athletes and the activities in which virtually all children participate—nonorganized sports and physical education classes.

In 1980 researchers from the Southern Illinois University School of Medicine offered some very important insights in a paper entitled "Sports-related Injuries in School-aged Children" (*The American Journal of Sports Medicine*, 8:5, 318–24, 1980). They studied all sports-related injuries at the fifty-three public and private schools in Springfield, Illinois, for one year and reported that nonorganized sports and physical education classes each produced nearly twice as many injuries as organized sports.

The sports with the highest incidence of injuries were football (19 percent of all injuries), basketball (15 percent), gym games (11 percent), baseball (10 percent), and roller skating (6 percent). The highest incidence of injuries for boys occurred at the age of fifteen (15 percent of all fifteen-year-old boys sustained an injury) and for girls at age fourteen (8 percent). Across all grades, boys sustained twice as many injuries as girls, although the school population was evenly divided between boys and girls.

The number one site of injury was the head, with fingers coming in a close second. Then in a dead heat for third place were knees and ankles. (Knees were the leading injury site in three sports: football, gymnastics, and track and field.) However, where 11 percent of the head injuries were considered "serious," fully 20 percent of the knee injuries were in that category.

By checking detailed descriptions of how the injuries were sustained, the investigators found that 27 percent were avoidable. By this they mean the injury was caused by recklessness, a lack of appropriate safety equipment, or some other factor that could easily have been avoided had the player taken minimal precautions. The same researchers recorded only one such avoidable injury during organized sports, but fully half of the injuries in physical education and nonorganized sports were caused by an inappropriate action on the part of the injured player. The researchers concluded, "These data strongly suggest the important role of adequate training, protective equipment, and supervision in injury avoidance.''

In a much smaller study, New York City investigators found that children's injuries in a nonorganized setting without adult supervision accounted for 41 percent of all injuries, suggesting that preventive and educational programs must be directed at the community as a whole and not just at organized sports programs.

And a 1983 review of the available literature (*The Physician and Sportsmedicine*, 11-7:1983, 116–22) found yet another factor that is contributing to the injury of young athletes: overuse.

Overuse injuries are chronic inflammatory conditions caused by repeated stress from excessive motion or impact shock. Many factors contribute to any given overuse injury but the end result of all of them is microtrauma. When microtrauma occurs there is no permanent damage. You'd literally need a microscope to see that there was any trauma at all. But when microtrauma is not allowed to heal, over time small microscopic injuries get bigger and bigger until finally—injury and pain.

Overuse injuries were once seen primarily in adults, the result of repetitive work or sports activities. Today it's the young athlete who is paying the price and a lot sooner than an adult would in comparable circumstances. There are a lot of reasons why kids are more susceptible to overuse injury. One of the most significant is that a youngster's body is not fully formed, not fully protected.

The child is most at risk during growth spurts. The muscle tendon unit that spans joints and bones becomes tighter during growth and even more so during growth spurts. This tightness can translate into a dramatic loss of flexibility, which spells trouble for an athlete whose body has to absorb a sudden force, such as during jumping or hurdling, or the repetitive strains of running or throwing. This increased risk of injury during growth spurts is well known to ballet teachers, who will often decrease the intensity of training during the growth spurts in order to avoid injury.

This is a good practice; the intensity of training should be reduced during periods of rapid growth. Unfortunately just the opposite is most likely to occur. For example, during the late summer when youngsters begin football practice, they may go from only a few hours of activity a week to six to eight hours of practice a day.

That is a dangerous situation. The healthiest game plan is to advance training by no more than 10 percent a week. This gives the body a chance to adapt to the demands of greater activity without hurting itself. And all of this also underscores the vital need youngsters have for flexibility training—no one seems to be showing youngsters how to stretch.

You can't detect a young athlete who's too tight by just looking at him or her, and there's little else you can tell at a glance about what these youngsters can or can't do. It's tempting to look at tall, adultlike bodies and forget that children live inside. I recall a fifteen-year-old basketball player, well over six feet tall, whose knees were so painfully swollen that it was a struggle for him just to get through the first half. His height and weight were those of an adult, but the muscles of his thighs were like those of a little boy.

Such discrepancies are not uncommon, yet we tend to lump kids together by calendar age, not developmental maturity. Such grouping totally ignores the fact that, at age six, maturity levels can vary as much as four years; by the age of twelve the difference can be as much as six years. One twelve-year-old may be developmentally closer to many sixteen-year-olds and ready for increased training and intense competition, while his twelve-year-old buddy may actually be closer physically to a nine-year-old and should be concentrating on developing basic skills and having fun.

How can you tell? Muscle definition is one factor in males. The kind of muscle definition that is thought of as the male physique—well-defined chest, arm, and leg muscles—require age-related hormones. Secondary sex characteristics may also be used to determine developmental maturity. For boys this means the development of facial hair, sometimes acne, and hair under the arms; for girls it is breast development and the onset of menses. Finally, an observer should be able to gauge competitive age by paying attention to overall coordination, specifically hand/eye coordination.

Let's also face the fact that kids (of all ages) often throw themselves into activity with more zeal than common sense. These kids don't know when to stop and will drive themselves unmercifully. I have seen kids drive their legs to the point where they actually break their bones, and they pound their joints until they've finally got a severe case of synovitis. I treated one wrestler with an immobilizing brace and eventually put him into a long leg cast because he refused to comply with doctor's orders to keep his knee immobile during recovery. But this boy was not to be stopped. Even the cast couldn't prevent him from running two to three miles a day!

Although the factors contributing to overuse injuries are, for the most part, not fully appreciated, one in particular may actually be *overemphasized*: anatomic malalignment. While it is true that leg-length discrepancies, flat feet, kneecap malalignments, and other skeletal variables may contribute to overuse injury, the body can adjust to a wide range of anatomic variables, *provided that changes in the patterns of physical activity are gradual.* I have seen patients with considerable malalignment who never seem to be bothered by structural problems. They had to proceed at a slower pace than their peers, perhaps, but their subsequent conditioning was not hampered in the least.

Because malalignment is so obvious, sometimes it gets blamed for problems it really hasn't caused. A child with "squinting patellae," or kneecaps that are off center and leaning toward the center of the body, could have a problem because of this slight malformation. However, if the youngster was advanced too quickly in basketball and this lead to "jumper's knee," there could be a misdiagnosis. Upon examination the doctor sees the malalignment and decides that's what caused the problem. In reality the child simply did too much too soon. Unfortunately, once the malalignment diagnosis has been made, the child could be treated for his "congential condition" or, worse, advised that sports are contraindicated. What should have happened? The youngster should have received proper treatment for his or her overuse problem, which would have meant rest, reduction of sporting activity, and changes in training technique.

The typical volunteer coach who is handling a Little League club or a Pop Warner football team probably has little knowledge about the prevention, recognition, and treatment of any type of injury, least of all an overuse injury. When this is combined with a child's natural enthusiasm in a competitive situation, injuries often occur. Remember, kids are kids, athletes or not.

Here's what must be done to lower the injury rates of young athletes:

1. Conditioning should be encouraged as a year-round goal, not just a seasonal chore. Although this is a bigger problem for young female athletes, too many guys also suffer from part-time conditioning. At the least, conditioning programs should be maintained throughout the season, not abandoned in favor of drills and scrimmages once the season is under way.

2. Accurate and extensive records need to be kept of each athlete's injury and fitness history. Unless records are kept, an accurate picture of each athlete's unique tendencies is difficult to establish.

3. Special attention needs to be paid to the knee in the preseason physical exam. Prevention is still the best treatment of knee injuries, and a careful examination can offer a lot of insight into the individual's risk of injury and how best to prevent it.

4. Training regimens should be specifically designed for young athletes who are physically, socially, and psychologically immature, not borrowed from programs designed for the mature athlete.

5. Parents must look at the athletic programs in their school districts and be sure that everything realistically possible is being done to ensure safety.

6. Schools should keep good records of sports-related injury and be able to compare their record of injury to national averages. In medicine this is called quality assurance. If there is a significant discrepancy, some serious deficiences may need to be addressed.

7. Respect the young athlete's limits. In unorganized play most children will not overload their systems to the point of injury. When there is pressure, however, from parents, community, and peers to practice long hours, compete, and win, undue stress on a developing body can cause temporary or even permanent injury.

8. During periods of rapid growth, intensity of training should be reduced and specific, slow, stretching exercises initiated in order to prevent injury.

9. The rate, duration, or intensity of training should not be increased more than 10 percent per week. A youngster running (pain-free) fifteen minutes a day, five days a week, could probably run safely seventeen minutes per day the following week. Likewise, a young swimmer managing 1,000 yards a day may be expected to safely advance to 1,100 yards per day the next week.

10. Shoes and equipment should fit. It can be expensive to continually replace outgrown equipment, but injuries are much more expensive. This is not *The Bad News Bears*. Youngsters don't need the most expensive or the most stylish equipment, but everything must fit.

11. Maintaining equipment is also very important. Air cells and fluid-filled sacs, for example, should be monitored in football helmets. Padding that's supposed to be soft and protective shouldn't be hard as a rock.

A lot of this is just good common sense, but our passion for sports, and especially for winning, is such in our culture that it's often easy to forgo common sense and just forge ahead. I sometimes wonder how such bright people—coaches, principals, teachers, doctors—can lose touch so quickly. A kid gets sent in for "just one more play" when he really can't take it, and then we act surprised when he's injured.

Sports and sporting activities are an integral part of growing up. We can't follow our children around or predict every stumble. But looking at today's injury rates makes it clear that we can do a lot more to protect our children.

Epilogue

Knee News Is Good News

Sports medicine is still a very young science: consider, for example, that the United States now has over 1,000 sports medicine clinics, up from just 300 in 1980. We really have only about ten years of experience with arthroscopy in this country—*The Journal of Arthroscopic and Related Surgery* was first published in 1985. This means that there are a lot of major advances ahead.

What's on the horizon for knees and knee owners? The two most promising areas of research involve two of the biggest pains in the knee: ligaments and cartilage.

REPLACING LIGAMENTS or TENDONS

Of all the formidable challenges in sports medicine, none are of the magnitude posed by the knee with an injury to the ligamentous support structure. These injuries often do not heal properly because the scar tissue that forms during the healing lacks the resiliency of the original ligament and prevents the recovery of full movement and stability. We've tried casting, bracing, and operating on these weakened knees. We've shaked them, baked them, and tried to rehabilitate them, yet still the search goes on for a satisfactory way to stabilize a wobbly knee.

One answer seems to be natural or artificial replacements for torn ligaments. One artificial ligament uses pure elemental carbon processed into long filaments and coated with an absorbable material that promotes ligament-forming cells to construct another ligament. After about six months the carbon begins to fragment, theoretically leaving behind newly grown ligamentous tissue that can function without the artificial support. Sometimes, though, the artificial support vanishes before the ligamentous tissue has had a chance to be strengthened by fibrous ingrowth. And there is some question as to whether the new tissue really can handle the demands that are placed upon it by an active life-style.

Another option is using the "natural" tendon of an animal that has been chemically processed to remove any components that might cause the body to reject this foreign tissue. Although the use of this material in the knee is still experimental, cardiac surgeons have been using it on heart-valve transplant recipients for fifteen years, so we're confident that there will be few problems with rejection. The process that is used to prevent rejection also greatly increases the strength and pliability of the tissue.

Two new developments also show promise. One is a synthetic fiber called Gore-Tex, which is basically the same material used in making raincoats. The six-inch artificial ligament looks like a braided rope with eyelets on either end that attach to the shin and thighbones with stainless-steel screws. Unlike the coated carbon fibers, Gore-Tex is designed as a permanent implant. It doesn't deform, it doesn't stretch out, and it's three times stronger than the human ligament it replaces. With most ligament reconstruction it takes a year before people can return to a nearly normal level of activity, but with Gore-Tex some patients are back to about 90 percent in about a month.

Collagen, which is used to make scars and wrinkles disappear, is another material that may help bolster the weak-kneed. This natural protein may soon be used to help "weave" tendons or ligaments back together so that they will heal.

At the University of Arizona researchers are stripping collagen of its cell-to-cell glue and then weaving it into a fabriclike band that can be wrapped around the injured ligament during surgery. Once in place, it acts like scaffolding, allowing the tendon or ligament to grow into it. Then, once the healing is complete, the collagen disappears.

All of these ligament replacements are so new that nobody knows whether they'll stand up to years and years of pressure and twisting. However, since 95 percent of the knees out there with instability significant enough to require surgery have little or no ACL left, we need to find some way to get support back into the knee. These approaches give hope to all the people who have given up sports as a result of ligamentous injuries.

REPLACING CARTILAGE

For individuals suffering cartilage damage, two new techniques may one day salvage or replace torn menisci. You may recall that the knee's shock absorbers have poor healing properties. Unlike most body tissue, the meniscus has a rich blood supply to only about its outer third, meaning that when the inner two thirds of the meniscus is torn, there is little or no healing. A new surgical technique creates channels from the outer rim of the meniscus to the inner portion, allowing blood and critical building materials to permeate the tissue.

The same research team which has given us meniscal channeling is also working on meniscal transplants. Cartilage cells are "immunologically privileged material," which means they are surrounded by a matrix that somehow protects them from rejection. Thus it is reasonable to suspect that someday we may be able to transplant a meniscus just like we now transplant full organs such as a heart or a kidney.

REBUILDING CARTILAGE

Another exciting strategy is rebuilding young joints biologically. The man who is helping surgery patients recover faster with his continuous passive-motion machine has a new technique that could save children from having to undergo artificial joint replacements.

Dr. Robert Salter is a professor of orthopedic surgery at the University of Toronto and senior orthopedic surgeon at the Hospital for Sick Children in Toronto. Young children are not considered suitable candidates for total knee replacement, since they would outlive the artificial knee by many decades, so he has been looking for a biological rather than a biomechanical means of rebuilding and restoring severely damaged knees.

What he has found is that a small graft of bone taken from a patient's tibia will form cartilage and not bone when it is surgically relocated and placed upside down in a diseased or damaged joint. In animal studies his biological resurfacing has completely restored the contour of severely damaged patellar grooves with tissue that is very comparable to smooth, intact knee cartilage. Part of the key to this technique, he says, is the use of his continuous passive motion after the surgery, which stimulates the growth of the graft. As we go to press Dr. Salter is ready to begin clinical trials with young patients.

NEW KNEE TECHNOLOGY FROM OLD

These new techniques will likely be joined by new ways of using old technology. Magnetic Resonance Imaging (MRI), for example, is giving us a new view of the injured knee. We mentioned earlier that MRI is likely to replace some standard knee tests as we learn how to use this incredible new tool. Already we're beginning to see things with MRI that we have not been able to see without opening up the knee. In fact, in some cases we're actually able to detect problems with MRI that we'd likely miss even if we did an arthroscopy. For example, researchers here in Southern California at Cedars-Sinai Medical Center are detecting fractures with MRI that are even invisible to X ray. The trick is that MRI can detect little drops of blood where they are not supposed to be: That means there's a fracture. The scientists at Cedars found that this new approach revealed a lot of heretofore unrecognized fractures. According to Dr. John Crues, director of Magnetic Resonance Imaging at Cedars-Sinai, "These occult fractures are a lot more common than we thought. They're extremely common, for example, among skiers who have had a tear of the collateral ligament." MRI can also reveal problems that are often mistaken for meniscal tears, and when there is a torn meniscus MRI can reveal the extent of damage better than any other imaging system.

Years ago we experimented with electrical and magnetic stimulation to speed healing. Now there are new pencil-thin, inch-and-a-half-long titanium batteries that may shorten recuperation time following surgery when they're placed alongside a newly recon-structed ligament or tendon. Canadian researchers report that the stimulator plus rehabilitation has gotten 40 percent of the athletes studied back into play—soccer, football, and hockey—in just twenty weeks. That's about twice as fast as one would expect.

These are just a few of the things that we know about. Research-ers are working on dozens of new procedures and refining older technologies that will keep those of us in sports medicine struggling to keep up with it all. In 1973 I began the first fellowship in the then brand-new field of sports medicine. At that time I knew this was an area of excitement and challenge that could benefit millions of people. We have traveled a great distance since then and have certainly accomplished a lot, but as I look ahead it seems evident that we've really just begun the trip.

Appendix A

Stretches and Exercises

STRETCHING TIPS

Improper stretching can injure the muscles being stretched.

Precede stretching exercises with a mild warm-up of whatever activity you're about to undertake.

Don't waste your time with calisthenics. They don't stretch your tight muscles, don't strengthen your weak ones, and don't even use your muscles in the same manner you will use them when you exercise.

Stretching should be slow and graceful.

Static stretching is done by bending, pushing, or pulling a body segment slowly and gently until a stretch is felt.

A stretch should not hurt but should produce a good feeling of mild tension.

Overstretching that is painful will actually produce tightness and possibly injury.

An easy, relaxed stretch should be held for thirty seconds.

Do not use ballistic stretches. The tension created during bouncing and bobbing is more than double that created during a slow gentle stretch and is enough to cause injury to your muscles and tendons.

If you have a physical condition that is aggravated by a certain movement, discontinue that movement and see a specialist.

Stretch before *and after* a workout.

If you tend to be tight-jointed, you should probably devote extra time to stretching and flexibility training to reduce the chance of muscle pulls.

It takes weeks to increase flexibility, but less time to lose flexibility. Therefore, a year-round stretching program is best.

EXERCISE TIPS

Approach your exercises in a progressive manner. Start with an easy routine and increase the number of exercises as your tolerance improves.

Each exercise session should start without weights. Weights are added gradually to your maximum effort, then reduced gradually as you move into a cooling-down period.

Every set of exercises should be followed by up to two minutes of complete relaxation to permit your tissues to receive an adequate supply of fresh blood and carry away waste products.

If you have a physical condition that is aggravated by a certain exercise, discontinue that exercise and see a specialist.

If you experience severe soreness from exercising, you have overdone the activity.

Grinding, pain, or a recurrence of swelling are signals that your exercise program is too aggressive and must be modified.

If you tend to be loose-jointed, you should probably concentrate on developing strength to avoid sprains.

WARNING: Squats or deep knee bends are one of the worst exercises you can inflict on an innocent knee. Forget them.

STRETCHING

A good flexibility program features a routine of between twelve and twenty-four exercises that stretch all major muscle groups. Some athletic trainers suggest what amounts to the basic yoga positions or slight variations. For example, Figure 1 is a good groin/inner thigh stretch that is akin to the "lotus" position. You should do this stretch with your back against a wall and a pillow in the small of your back. You can do two different stretches from this position. First, put the bottoms of your feet together, then pull your heels toward your groin as you move your upper body forward. Then, with your feet together and pulled as close to your buttocks as possible, push down on your knees. (For all of these stretches work up to where you can repeat them five to ten times.) If this stretch is too painful,

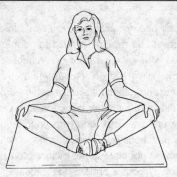

Figure 1

you can work up to it by adjusting your feet for comfort. Move your feet
farther from your buttocks or, if necessary, cross your feet.

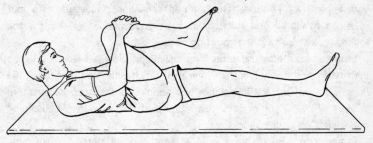

Figure 2

Pain behind your knee is often caused by tight hamstrings. The hamstring stretch (Figure 2) may help relieve this pain and it will help prevent
injury. Lie on the floor or some other firm surface. (We say this because if

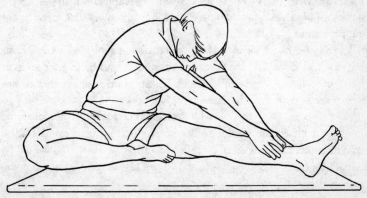

Figure 3

you try this on a water bed, for example, you could fold up like a cot.) Pull your knee to your chest and raise your head to your knee. Eventually you should be able to kiss your knee, which is one rehabilitative effort we never discussed. Who know? It worked on scrapes when you were a child.

Another good hamstrings stretch is shown in Figure 3. From the position shown, grab your ankle and pull your body forward. Obviously if you can't grab your ankle the first time out, don't rip your seams trying. For all of these stretches, the directions give you an idea of what you need to be working *toward* if you're not already the picture of flexibility.

Although not shown, your standard toe touch is also good for the hamstrings. Keep your heels together and knees straight. (If, from this position, you can't even *see* your feet, a good weight-loss program is also certainly in order.) The object is to try to touch the ground or floor with your fingers. Don't bounce! That's not only cheating, it's hazardous to your muscular health. If you suffer lower-back problems, better skip the toe touches or risk aggravating your bad back.

Some athletes also use something called the plow, where they lie on their backs and throw their legs over their heads until their toes touch the floor. This stretches the hamstrings and brings countless new patients into doctors' offices. If you're going to use the plow, brace yourself by keeping your hands on your buttocks.

Runners, in particular, are fond of another killer stretch. They enjoy walking up to a wall and throwing one leg up against it. With one leg extended ninety degrees or more, these runners have a high chance of injury using this exercise. Although it looks innocent enough (as opposed to the plow, which looks like it could maim a contortionist), this is a very advanced stretch and should be excluded from almost all athletic conditioning programs.

Leaving the hams, we move on to the quadriceps muscles. Grab a chair but don't sit down (Figure 4). Stand up straight and bend your knee to bring your heel toward your buttock. Grasp your ankle as shown and slowly move your thigh backward and hips forward while maintaining an upright position. (Now you see why the chair is necessary.) The same basic front-thigh stretch can be done while you're lying on your stomach. The advantage here is, you can lift and stretch both legs at once. That would be a real trick from a standing position. You can also do one leg at a time by resting on one elbow.

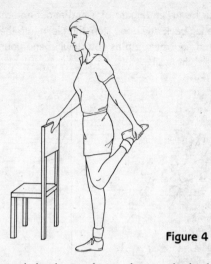

Figure 4

Figure 5 is a good stretch for the quadriceps, but it is *for healthy knees only!* This stretch is done at more of an angle out from the midline of the body than the preceding stretches and thus puts more pressure on your knee. This could be painful. If it is, leave this one alone until you've recovered. If performed correctly, a healthy knee should enjoy this one. Lie on your back with your knee up and leg pulled into your side, then slowly lower your knee.

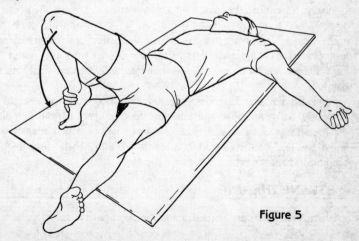

Figure 5

For your lower leg (Figure 6), stand about an arm's length from a wall. Move one leg back one good step, then lean into the wall. Keep your back foot flat and your head up as you slowly bend your arms and lower your body toward the wall.

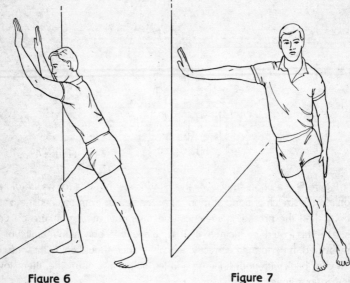

Figure 6   **Figure 7**

Finally, it's time to do something for your knee stabilizers, the abductor muscles, and your iliotibial band (Figure 7). Stand one arm's length from a wall. Move the leg closest to the wall back and behind your other leg. Your foot should be behind and off to the far side of your other foot. Lean into the wall several inches until you feel that your abductors are tight (but not painful).

Obviously you should repeat these stretches using both legs. And just as obviously, we're not offering a total stretching program here. Doing all of these stretches on a regular basis, however, will help you protect your knees and lead you naturally into a rehabilitative or general strengthening program, which is next.

STRENGTHENING

We're going to start out assuming that your leg muscles have been severely weakened. However, even if you're lucky enough to have some solid muscular support, this first exercise, done several times a day, can be invaluable for rebuilding your quadriceps muscles. Remember: These are the critical muscles that, if weakened, can in and of themselves cause knee problems. For example, if you have arthritis, strengthening your quadriceps muscles may take a load off of your knee and substantially decrease your pain.

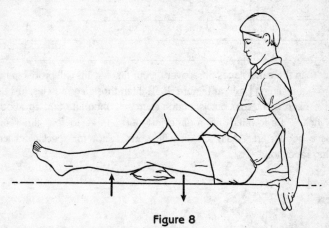

Figure 8

This terrific quads builder is a simple isometric exercise (Figure 8). Place a rolled towel under the small of your knee; the idea is to keep your knee joint straight. Tighten the muscles in your leg, without moving your knee, and hold that contraction. (You may want to help tighten your hamstring muscles by pointing your toes toward your knee.) Work up to where you can keep those muscles taut for at least thirty seconds, then relax and repeat up to twenty-five times. You can do this exercise several times a day. Some people recommend repeating it every hour during the initial stages of recovery. Of course if you're just out of surgery or recovering from a serious injury or muscular disorder, follow your doctor's orders regarding how often and how many repetitions are best for you. If you are rehabilitating an old injury, this exercise can (and should) be done dozens of times a day. You don't have to keep your legs straight, so you can do it while you're working at a desk, eating dinner, watching television, or while doing any of a dozen or more similar activities throughout your day. This is an especially good exercise if you have chondromalacia patella.

Figure 9

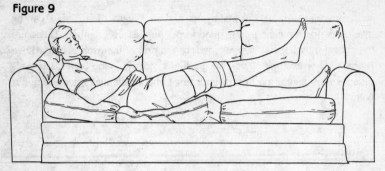

If you're in the early stages of recovery, your first leg lifts will probably be done from a reclining position (Figure 9). Tighten those leg muscles, just as you have been doing for your isometric exercises, then lift your leg about twelve inches. Performing this routine just once, three to four times an hour, is a good start. Again, check with your doctor for specific advice regarding repetitions.

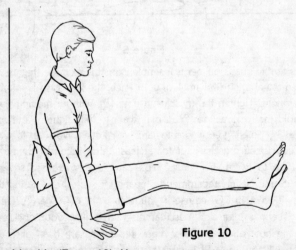

Figure 10

Standard leg lifts (Figure 10), like isometric contractions, are extremely important for rehabilitating the weak-kneed. Here's the best way to do leg lifts. Start with your back to a wall and a pillow in the small of your back. This is important, because you don't want your pelvic and back muscles to be lifting your leg. Also, if you have a problem with lower-back pain, this shouldn't aggravate it. Next use what we call the "Rule of Fives": Do your isometric contraction for a count of five, then raise your leg five inches, hold for another count of five, then lower your leg and relax for a count of five. Work up to doing three sets of ten, resting a couple of minutes between sets. Once you can do this with *both* legs, even your uninjured one, and you can do it without your leg quivering like Jell-O, you're ready for some weight resistance exercises.

Here's an all-purpose strengthener that lets one leg be the "weight" for the other: Sit back on a table or on a bed with your thigh supported all the way out to the knee. Cross your legs at your ankles and press the heel of one leg into the ankle of the other. Press down as hard as you can for thirty seconds. Relax, then repeat ten times for each leg. *(For all the subsequent exercises, work toward a goal of two to three sets of ten lifts each unless otherwise noted.)* Eventually, from a regular seated position, you can cross your legs, again at the ankles, and use one leg to lift the other. When you start out you can let your upper leg do a little work and help lift itself, but once you're on the road to recovery, this is cheating.

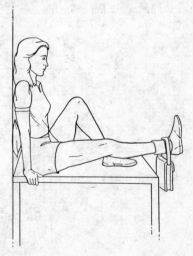

Figure 11

When it's time to move into weight resistant exercises, you can also use ankle weights if you have them, otherwise you can use a purse with a strap (Figure 11). If you don't even have access to a purse, try a sandwich bag filled with sand and tied into a sock. (We want no excuses here!) Start with straight-leg lifts with one or two pounds attached to each ankle and work up to about ten pounds. Once you're at that level, it's easier if you can spend a little time with weight training equipment, but don't try to do too much too soon. Here's one way to avoid that: Find a starting point for each exercise. This is whatever weight you can lift ten times with the last few times being somewhat of a strain. For each exercise do your first ten lifts as briskly as you can. Then reduce the weight by several pounds and repeat, for a total of three or four sets. At first, three sets may be a real challenge, but as you get stronger, add on sets, not weights. You may increase your starting weight if you want, but reduce that weight by ten to twenty pounds for subsequent sets. Never emphasize lifting impressive loads of steel; leave that to the iron pumpers trying to sculpt the perfect body. You should simply be aiming for healthy knees that won't send you into early sports retirement.

When you start with the weighted leg lifts keep your leg straight, and thus your knee protected. (Such straight-leg lifts are another especially valuable exercise for chondromalacia sufferers.) You then graduate to bent-leg ankle lifts (Figure 12). Don't bend your knee yet, just bend your ankle and exercise important lower leg muscles.

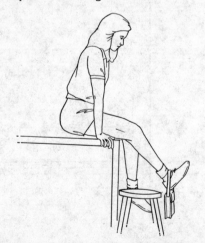

Figure 12

Eventually try leg lifts from this position, but be careful. If you have chondromalacia, for example, you need to have built up your muscles with all the preceding exercises before starting this routine. In fact, if you want to be real good to your knees, prop your leg up on a stool or chair from your position in Figure 12. Before you lift a pound you want your leg two thirds of the way toward full extension (out straight).

The problem is that when your leg is bent as it is in Figure 12, those first few degrees of movement to lift your leg create the greatest forces across your knee. So when doing weighted bent-leg lifts, you want to avoid this extra stress. Fortunately just lifting a weight across those last fifteen to twenty degrees of extension will help strengthen your muscles.

For your abductor and adductor muscles, which run alongside your lower leg, press your foot against one side of a solid object and then the other side of your foot (Figure 13). If you don't happen to have a cement cinder block handy, the side of a heavy table leg will do nicely.

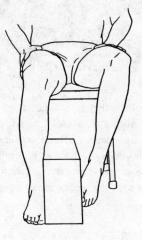

Figure 13

ADVANCED EXERCISES

Once you've done all of the above, you're ready for some final refinement. Since we were just working on abductors and adductors, you can use ankle weights (or your now handy purse or sandy sock) and try side lifts (Figure 14). Lie on your side, legs straight, one arm under your head and the other on the floor in front of your chest for support. Slowly raise your leg about forty-five degrees, then lower it to the floor without touching the floor. This works your abductors. For your adductors (Figure 15), place one leg on a chair, slowly lift your other leg to meet it, then return it slowly to the floor.

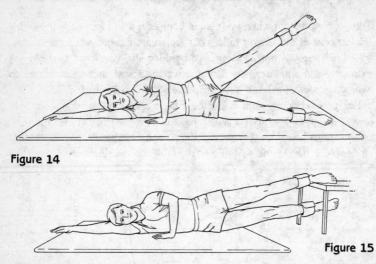

Figure 14

Figure 15

Next, for your hamstrings (Figure 16), lie on your stomach, chin to the floor, with your ankle weights still in place. Slowly lift one leg six to twelve inches, then lower it just as slowly, without touching the floor. You can do this same exercise with your knee bent as you raise only your lower leg, but again bent-knee exercises put extra pressure across a kneecap, so make sure your knee is in pretty healthy shape before even trying this one.

Figure 16

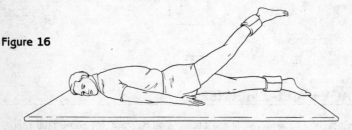

Finally, for those quads that are crucial for happy knees, do a wall sit (Figure 17). Stand three feet from a wall, lean back against it, and squat until your legs are perpendicular to the wall. To anyone walking in on your exercise, you'll look like you're sitting on an invisible chair. (Of course it's cheating to actually use one.) Hold this position for thirty seconds. Build up to a set of five two-minute wall sits. For those millions of people weak-kneed because of significant quadriceps deficiencies, this one exercise can be a real knee saver.

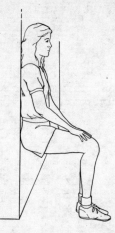

Figure 17

And for the well-healed who are now looking for some fine-tuning, you can hop to it (Figure 18). Jump side to side over an object. You can start with a big-city phone book for a three- to four-inch obstacle, gradually moving up to a small footstool or similar object of about one foot in height. This exercise helps develop power, balance, and agility. Jump rapidly from side to side until fatigue develops or your downstairs neighbors complain.

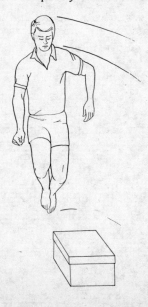

Figure 18

Appendix B

Glossary of Orthopedic and Sports Medicine Terms

Abduction: To move a limb or any other part away from the midline, or center, of the body.

Adduction: To move a limb or any other part toward the midline, or center of the body.

Anterior: Toward the front of the body.

Anterior cruciate ligament: The ACL and the posterior cruciate ligament cross inside the knee joint and provide the knee with vital strength and stability.

Anterior drawer test: One of several simple tests for knee stability that detects damage to the anterior cruciate ligament.

Arthrogram: Used primarily to detect meniscal tears, this diagnostic test involves injecting an anesthetized knee joint with a contrast dye (or air) that can be seen by X ray.

Arthroscope: An instrument for viewing and, if necessary, operating on the interior of a joint using a fiber-optic light source and a thin flexible tube that contains a miniature video system.

Bursitis: Inflammation of any of the fluid-containing sacs (bursa) that provide cushioning for tendons around joints, including the knees, heels, shoulders, and elbows.

CAT, or "C.T.," scan: Computerized axial tomography is a sophisticated form of X ray that is 100 times as sensitive as an ordinary X ray and takes a cross-sectional view of the body.

Cartilage: To alleviate bone-on-bone wear and tear, nature covers the ends of active bones with this dense, elastic connective tissue that acts as a natural shock absorber. (See MENISCUS.)

Chondromalacia patella (also known as "runner's knee") Degeneration or softening of the cartilage in the kneecap (patella) caused by overuse or malalignment.

Condyles: Eliptical notches at the ends of major bones. The condyles of the femur are associated with a condition known as iliotibial band friction syndrome.

Cybex (trademark): A finely calibrated rehabilitation exercise machine capable of detecting and documenting subtle differences in muscular strengths.

Debridement: This surgical technique has been compared to "mowing the lawn." Rough spots of cartilage are shaved off and the irritating pieces are then whisked away by irrigating the knee.

Dislocation: Displacement of bones meeting at a joint. Bones are restored to their normal position by manipulation, which may require local or general anesthesia (See SUBLUXATION.)

Effusion: Popularly, effusion is equated with general swelling; technically, effusion is swelling within a joint caused by a fluid such as blood escaping into the body cavity.

Epiphyseal fracture: A rupture or crack of the growth plate of long bones. This plate (epiphysis) fuses to the bone with skeletal maturity.

Extension: Straightening of a joint.

Femur: The "thighbone" is one of the three bones making up the knee joint. It is the largest bone in the body, originating at the pelvis.

Flexion: Bending of a joint.

Fracture: A break, rupture, or crack in a bone or cartilage.

Gout: An inflammation of the joints produced by an excess of uric acid, a by-product of normal metabolism, which leads to the formation of needle-sharp crystals of monosodium urate in the joints.

Hamstring muscles: Often neglected in exercise, these muscles run along the back of the leg and are responsible for flexing the knee.

Iliotibial band friction syndrome: An inflammatory condition caused by the irritation of the muscle group known as the iliotibial band, which stretches over the end of the femur.

Isometric exercise: Fixed muscular contraction that does not involve any movement of the joint or limb.

-itis: A suffix indicating inflammation.

Kneecap: See PATELLA.

Lachman test: One of several simple tests to check for knee stability, this one is considered more sensitive than the anterior drawer test and determines cruciate ligament integrity.

Lateral: Away from the midline, or center, of the body.

Ligaments: Strong, fibrous tissue that links two bones together at a joint. Collateral ligaments run up the inside and outside of the leg. The cruciate ligaments cross with the joint. (See SPRAIN.)

Magnetic resonance imaging: MRI is a diagnostic technology that uses a superconducting magnet and a computer to precisely image internal soft body tissue.

McMurray's test: One of several simple tests to detect knee stability, this one specifically checks for meniscal damage.

Medial: Toward the midline, or center, of the body.

Meniscectomy: Once the most common knee surgery, the complete removal of the knee's meniscus has been replaced by a partial meniscectomy, which removes as little of the damaged meniscus as possible to provide continued protection of the knee.

Meniscus: A crescent-shaped structure that divides the cavity of synovial joints, such as between the thigh and leg bones at the knee, and provides shock absorption. Although commonly used as a synonym for "cartilage," they're not anatomically the same.

Non-steroidal anti-inflammatory drugs: NSAIDS, as they are called, *may* have fewer side effects and require fewer doses than the "gold standard" of all inflammation fighters, aspirin.

Orthopedics: A medical specialty that deals with treatment and prevention of disorders of the musculoskeletal system, which includes bones, muscles, joints, ligaments, tendons, and related structures.

Orthotics: These devices straighten or balance your foot in its neutral position, thereby relieving extra pressures caused by inherently unbalanced feet. Although some over-the-counter orthotics are available, the most effective are medically prescribed and made from a cast of your foot.

Osgood-Schlatter's disease (also known as "football" or "rugby knee"): Although its exact cause is unknown, this painful condition appears to be associated with the immaturity of the growth plate at the front end of the tibia and is most often associated with vigorous sporting activities.

Osteoarthritis: The most common form of arthritis is a disease of joint cartilage, which is secondary to underlying bone damage, usually an old injury.

Osteochondritis dissecans: A condition that causes a small area of bone (usually at the end of the femur) to degenerate or become necrotic, causing a small but painful lesion. Small bone fragments may actually break away and go floating around the knee joint.

Osteotomy: This major surgical procedure changes the alignment of your knees by removing a small wedge of bone, usually from the outer side of the knee, in order to more evenly distribute pressure across the knee.

Overuse injury: Trauma caused by repeated stress to tissue from excessive motion or impact shock.

Patella: Also known as the kneecap, the patella is the protective bone at the front of the knee and one of three bones that make up the knee joint.

Patellofemoral: Associated with the patella and the track it moves in plus the femur.

Patellar tendinitis: A microscopic tear of the tendons connecting the kneecap to the thigh muscles and shinbone causes this condition, which is also known as "jumper's knee." It's usually sports related and represents an overuse of these tendons.

Plicae: These are developmental leftovers of the membrane walls that organize a developing knee. They are supposed to disappear toward the end of fetal development, but often pieces remain and they can irritate an innocent knee.

Posterior: Toward the back of the body.

Posterior cruciate ligament: See ANTERIOR CRUCIATE LIGAMENT.

Pronation: Ankles can excessively roll either inward or outward. The most common is pronation, in which the ankles roll inward, causing extra pressures on many of the muscles and bones of the feet, legs, and knees. (See SUPINATION.)

Pseudo-locking: The knee is not actually blocked from closing (locking) or incapable of complete movement, but some movements simply hurt too much to do, giving the impression of a locked knee.

Pseudo-gout: An inflammatory condition resembling gout, caused by crystals of calcium pyrophosphate in the synovial membrane and fluid. Diagnosis is made by examining the synovial fluid.

Quadriceps: A group of four major anterior thigh muscles that are involved in knee joint extension and which weaken quickly with knee injury.

Rehabilitation: Reconditioning of the musculoskeltal system to restore maximum function.

Rheumatologist: A medical doctor who specializes in rheumatic diseases such as arthritis.

Rheumatoid arthritis: The second most common form of arthritis, RA is an inflammatory condition of the joint lining and tends to be systemic, which means once you've got RA it may crop up in any joint or other body tissue.

Runner's knee: See CHONDROMALACIA PATELLA.

Soft, or low-impact, aerobics: Side-to-side marching, dance-walk combinations, or gliding movements are substituted for the jolting up-and-down motion of typical aerobic routines, which could make this form of aerobics safer.

Sprain: A break or tear in a ligament.

Stress X ray: Multiple X rays taken while the joint or bones are lightly moved and stressed.

Subluxation: Partial dislocation of bones at a joint. The bones return to their normal position without assistance.

Supination: Sometimes ankles will roll toward the outside of the body, and this condition, known as supination, causes extra pressures for the feet, legs, and knees. (See PRONATION.)

Synovial fluid: When someone says they have "water on the knee" it's really this thick, colorless lubricating fluid that is contained in a joint or a bursa. When the body pumps out too much synovial fluid, trying to manage an injury, there is swelling.

Tendon: A fibrous cord of connective tissue that attaches muscles to bone.

Tendinitis: Inflammation of a tendon.

"The terrible triad": A major injury to the knee, usually involving a rupture of the anterior cruciate ligament, the medial meniscus, and the medial collateral ligament.

Tibia: The larger of the two lower leg bones, the tibia is one of three bones that make up the knee.

Total joint replacement: A major surgery that replaces the patella, as well as the damaged ends of the femur and tibia, with metal and plastic surfaces in order to decrease pain and improve function.

Water on the knee: See SYNOVIAL FLUID.

It Certainly Doesn't End Here

As we have noted throughout this book, the field of sports medicine is changing so fast that in the time it has taken to get this book into your hands a number of important advancements have occurred. In order to keep you up to date on what you and your knees need to know, we invite you to subscribe to *Knee News and Sports Medicine*. This bimonthly newsletter will cover problems and symptoms, sports and activities, relief and rehabilitation for knees everywhere. To subscribe, mail a check or money order for $18.00 to:

Orthopedic Press
18034 Ventura Blvd.
Suite 311
Encino, CA 91316

(Outside of the United States, please add $2.00)

(To get a free copy of *Knee News and Sports Medicine*, send a #10 business-sized envelope with one ounce of postage and your address on the envelope to the above address.)

Index

Abductor muscles, 264, 269
Accreditation Association of Ambulatory
    Health Care (AAHC), 68
Acetaminophen, 82–83
Achilles' tendinitis, 159
Acute knee problems, 41–53
    acute meniscal tears, 8, 41–44, 50
    degenerative meniscal tears, 8, 44
    fractures, 50–53
    ligament tears (sprained knee),
        44–49
    terrible triad, 49–50
Acute meniscal tears, 8, 41–44, 50
Adductor muscles, 269
Aerobic dance, 4, 26, 168–175
    body check, 169
    common injuries, 172–173
    injury rates, 168–169
    shoes, 171
    soft aerobics, 171, 173–175
    tips for, 175
    training and conditioning, 169–171
Aerobic exercise, 128–130
    (See also Aerobic dance)
Aging athletes, 222–225
Alcoholics, 83
American Athletic Union, 241
American Board of Orthopedic Surgery,
    65
American College of Obstetrics and
    Gynecology, 175
American College of Sports Medicine,
    174
Analgesic creams, 84
Anatomic malalignment, 245
Anderson Knee Stabler, 123
Ankle weights, 112, 179–180, 267–269
Anterior cruciate ligament (ACL), 7–9,
    17, 24, 44, 45, 47–50, 71,
    88–89, 119, 184–185, 192–193
Anterior drawer test, 71–72
Anti-inflammatory drugs, 18, 27, 33,
    34, 36, 38, 80–84, 131–132
Apprehension sign, 31, 235
Arches, 140
Arthritis, 8, 9, 18, 31, 39, 54–59
    defined, 55–58
    diagnosis of, 58–59
    emotions and, 131
    exercise and, 126–131

football and, 195–196
    incidence of, 54
    medication and, 131–133
    osteoarthritis, 9, 21, 32, 54–56, 94,
        125, 126, 132–134
    rest and, 126
    rheumatoid, 55, 56–57, 97, 98, 125,
        126, 131–133
    surgery and, 133–135
Arthrogram, 74, 233
Arthrography, 59, 233
Arthroscope, 75, 90–91
Arthroscopy, 16, 21, 28, 38, 47, 59,
        75–77, 90–95, 116, 233
    arthritis and, 133–134
    combined with open surgery, 94, 95
    compared to open surgery, 91
    complications, 92–93
    incidence of, 87
Arthrotomy (see Surgery)
Artificial knees, 17, 96–99, 134–135
Artificial ligaments, 251–253
Aspirin, 18, 27, 36, 38, 80–82, 131–132

Ballet, 241, 243
Baseball, 242
Basketball, 4, 8, 11–14, 34, 189–194,
        238, 239, 241, 242
    body check, 190–191
    common injuries, 191–193
    conditioning, 191
    tips for, 193–194
Benoit, Joan, 95
Bicycling, 35, 187–188, 201–206, 238
    bike fitting, 203–204
    body check, 202–203
    common injuries, 204–206
    tips for, 206
Bindings, ski, 176, 180–183, 186
Biofeedback, 110
Biogen, Inc., 133
Body weight, 9, 105, 126, 127
Bone scan (radionuclide bone
        scintigraphy), 51
Boots, ski, 177, 183–184
Boston Children's Hospital, 240
Bowlegs, 156, 202
Boxing, 242
Braces, 28, 32, 34, 46, 98–99,
        102–103, 118–123

Braces, *(continued)*
  functional, 119–120
  prophylactic, 121–123
  rehabilitative, 120–121
  wraps, 118, 123–124
Breaststroker's knee, 212–213
Broad jump, 239
Broken bones, 50–52
Brooks shoes, 144
Bursa, 8, 32–33, 205, 208, 219
Bursitis (housemaid's knee), 8, 32–33,
    145, 164, 205, 210, 219

Calf muscles, 11
Calisthenics, 152–153
Cants, 178
Car-accident injuries, 4
Carter, Gary, 4
Cartilage, 8–9, 20, 23, 28, 55, 92–94, 134
  (See also Meniscus)
CAT scans (computerized axial
    tomography), 75
Cedars-Sinai Medical Center, 254
Center for Sports Medicine, San
    Francisco, 168–170, 172, 189
Children, 18, 229–247
  chondromalacia patella, 236–237
  epiphyseal injury, 199, 229,
    237–239
  Osgood-Schlatter's disease, 34, 199,
    230–231
  osteochondritis dissecans, 232–233
  patella dislocation/subluxation,
    234–236
  patellofemoral syndrome, 229–230,
    233–234
  sports, 238–247
Chondromalacia patella (runner's
    knee), 13, 21, 23, 24, 26–29,
    94, 157, 159–162, 172, 193,
    205, 213, 215, 236–237,
    265, 268
Chronic knee problems, 26–40
  bursitis (housemaid's knee), 8,
    32–33, 145, 164, 205, 210, 219
  chondromalacia patella (runner's
    knee), 13, 21, 23, 24, 26–29,
    94, 157, 159–162, 172, 193,
    205, 213, 215, 236–237,
    265, 268
  iliotibial band friction syndrome, 24,
    35–36, 145, 156, 159,
    162–163
  patellar tendinitis (jumper's knee),
    11, 33–35, 164, 172–173,
    192, 215

  patella subluxation (dislocated
    kneecap), 22, 29–32, 193,
    234–236
  Pathological Synovial Plicae, 36–38
  spontaneous osteonecrosis, 39–40
Closed manipulation, 115–116
Collagen, 252
Collateral ligaments, 6, 44, 94
Conditioning, 14, 15, 147–154
  aerobic dance, 168–171
  basketball, 191
  football, 197–199
  running, 158
  skiing, 179–180, 186
  wrestling, 208–209
  (See also Exercises)
Condyles, 35
Continuous passive motion (CPM), 98,
    253, 254
Cooper, Kenneth, 241
Corticosteroids, 132
Cortisone, 33, 76–77, 132
Crepitation, 23
Cross-country skiing, 185–187
Cruciate ligaments, 6–7, 71–73, 93–94
  anterior, 7–9, 17, 24, 44, 45, 47–50,
    71, 88–89, 119, 184–185,
    192–193
  posterior, 7, 44, 71, 120
Crues, John, 254
C.Ti. brace, 120
Cybex machine, 73, 111
Cycling *(see* Bicycling)

Dance, 4, 11, 26, 34, 35, 241, 243
  (See also Aerobic dance)
Dean, Dizzy, 218
Debridement, 93, 134
Degenerative meniscal tears, 44
Diagnostic tests, 66–67, 74–75
Dislocation, 22, 29–32, 193, 234–236
Doctors, choice of, 63–66
Downhill running, 163, 164
Downhill skiing, 176–177, 187
Drake seven-count straight-leg raise,
    106

Effusion, 17–19, 76
Elbow injuries, 217–219
Electrical Muscle Stimulation (EMS), 110
Electromedicine, 109–111
Endurance training, 179
Epiphyseal injury, 199, 200, 229,
    237–239
Esposito, Phil, 4
Estwanik, Joseph, 208

Exercises, 28, 34, 36, 38, 39, 43, 44,
52
advanced, 269–271
arthritis and, 126–131
calisthenics, 152–153
childrens' injuries and, 230, 234
functional, 128–129
isometric, 28, 106, 129, 151–152,
234, 265
range-of-motion, 28, 128
rehabilitative, 105–108
strengthening, 128, 129–130, 151,
158, 264–269
stretching, 14, 15, 148–150,
259–264
(See also Conditioning; Rehabilitation)

Feet, 139–146, 245
Femur, 6, 8, 13, 29, 35
Figure skating, 4
Flat feet, 245
Flexibility, 13, 148–150, 198, 244
Flexion contracture, 126
Football, 3, 4, 122, 188, 189,
195–200, 238, 241–244, 247
arthritis and, 195–196
common injuries, 199–200
conditioning, 197–199
Football/rugby knee (Osgood-Schlatter's
disease), 34, 199, 230–231
Fractures, 50–53
Functional braces, 119–120
Functional exercises, 128–129

Gender, injuries and, 12–15, 156, 157,
162, 168, 192–193, 202–
204
Germantown Medical Center, 131
Gibbs, Alex, 122
Giving way (see Dislocation; Subluxation)
Gold salts, 132, 133
Golf, 209–212
body check, 209–210
common injuries, 210–211
tips for, 211–212
Gore-Tex, 252
Gout, 18, 33, 55, 57, 125, 126
Great Plains Sports Medicine Founda-
tion, 216
Gymnastics, 3, 241, 242

Hamstring muscles, 11, 148, 150, 151,
159, 170, 179, 261–262, 270
Heart disease, 125
Hemarthrosis, 17, 92
Henning, Dan, 122

Highgenboten, Carl, 237
High jump, 239
High tibial osteotomy, 40, 97
Hippocrates, 80
Hockey, 238
Housemaid's knee (bursitis), 8, 32–33,
145, 164, 205, 210, 219
Hurdling, 11, 34
Hydrotherapy, 112–113, 129, 130
Hypnosis, 131

Ibuprofen, 83–84
Ice, 17–18, 34, 36, 38, 46, 130–131
Ice hockey, 188
Iliotibial band friction syndrome (IBFS),
24, 35–36, 145, 156, 159,
162–163
Interferon, 133
Internal bleeding, 17, 18
Internal derangement of the knee
(I.D.K.), 199
Isometric exercises, 28, 106, 129,
151–152, 234, 265

Jackson, Douglas, 157
Jefferson Medical College, 131
Jogging (see Running)
Jumper's knee (patellar tendinitis), 11,
24, 33–35, 164, 172–173,
192, 215

Kidney damage, 84, 85
King, Bernard, 4
Kneecap (patella), 9
(See also specific injuries)
Knee instability, 163
Knee News, 281
Knock knees, 156, 202
Kolin, Michael, 204

Lachman test, 73
Lactic acid, 150
Lane, Nancy, 156
Lateral femoral condyle, 162
Laternal step-up routine, 107
Lavage, 134
Leach, Robert E., 165
Leg curls, 214
Leg-length discrepancy, 156–157, 163,
245
Leg lifts, 266–269
Lenox Hill derotation brace, 99,
118–120
Levy, Allen, 197
Ligament replacements, 251–253

Ligaments, 6–8, 13, 17, 24, 229, 237–239
(See also Collateral ligaments; Cruciate ligaments)
Ligament tears (sprained knee), 44–49, 192–193
Locking, 20–21
Lupus, 57–58

Machine conditioning, 152
Magnetic resonance imaging (MRI), 51, 59, 66, 74–75, 254
Manipulation, 115–116
Mantle, Mickey, 3
Marino, Dan, 4
Massage, 109
McDavid Knee Guard, 123
McMurray's test, 71
Medial collateral ligament (MCL), 45, 47, 50, 184
Medial femoral condyle, 232
Medicare certification, 68
Meniscectomy, 8–9, 42–43
Meniscus, 8, 17, 20, 24, 25, 31
acute tears, 8, 41–44, 50
degenerative tears, 8, 44
diagnosis of tears, 74
surgery, 8–9, 42–43, 93, 253–254
Metcalf, Robert, 92
Methodist Hospital of Indiana, 216
Milo of Croton, 106
Muscles, 11, 14, 25, 105
(See also specific muscles)
Muscle spasms, 25

Namath, Joe, 3, 118
National Athletic Trainers' Association, Inc. (NATA), 14, 197
National Collegiate Athletic Association, 4
Needle aspiration, 18, 76
New Balance shoes, 144
Nicholas, James, 73
Nike, 144
Non-steroidal anti-inflammatory drugs, 80–84, 132
Northwestern University Medical School, 12, 13

Occupational Safety and Health Administration, 195
Orr, Bobby, 3
Orthotics, 34, 36, 140, 145–146, 159, 161, 173, 178, 219
Osgood-Schlatter's disease (football/rugby knee), 34, 199, 230–231

Osteoarthritis, 9, 21, 32, 54–56, 94, 125, 126, 132–134
Osteochondritis dissecans, 232–233
Osteotomy, 40, 97, 134
Overuse injuries, 216–217, 243–245

Pagliano, John, 157
Pain, 24, 25, 70, 71
acetaminophen and, 82–83
aspirin and, 18, 27, 36, 80–82, 131–132
creams and lotions and, 84
ibuprofen and, 83–84
physical therapy and, 114–115
psychological component of, 79–80
Panush, Richard, 155
Patellar tendinitis (jumper's knee), 11, 24, 33–35, 164, 172–173, 192, 215
Patella subluxation (dislocated knee-cap), 22, 29–32, 193, 234–236
Patellofemoral syndrome (anterior knee pain), 193, 229–230, 233–234
Pathological Synovial Plicae, 36–38
Pes anserinus, 164
Peterson, Cary, 204
Physical exmaination, 70–74, 242
Physical therapy, 108–116
Placebo effect, 85
Platelets, 81
Plicae, 36–38, 164
Plow, 262
Pole vault, 239
Popliteal tendinitis, 163–164
Posterior cruciate ligament (PCL), 7, 44, 71, 120
Prepatellar bursitis, 207–208
President's Council on Physical Fitness and Sports, 147, 241
Pronation, 139–140, 146, 159
Prophylactic braces, 121–123
Prostaglandins, 81
Pseudo-gout, 18
Pseudo-locking, 20, 21

Quadriceps muscles, 11, 13, 28, 31, 34, 129, 148, 151, 158, 159, 162, 170, 172, 179, 186, 231, 234, 235, 262–263, 265, 270

Racket sports, 3, 4, 35, 217–221
body check, 218–219
common injuries, 219–220
tips for, 221

Range-of-motion exercises, 28, 128
Rectifying-demodulating phono-
    pneumograph (RDP), 59
Rehabilitation, 69, 78, 89, 100–117
    exercises, 105–108
    keys to, 105
    non-surgical, 102–103
    old injuries, 103–105
    physical therapy, 108–116
    surgical, 101–102
    tips for, 116–117
Rehabilitative braces, 120–121
Rest, arthritis and, 126
Retton, Mary Lou, 95
Rhea, Jerry, 197
Rheumatoid arthritis, 55, 56–57, 59,
    97, 98, 125, 126, 131–133
Rheumatoid factor, 58
Rheumatologist, 58
RICE (rest, ice, compression, and
    elevation), 17–18, 46
Rippe, James, 144
Robinson, John, 144
Rockport Walking Institute, 144
Roller skating, 242
Rowing, 152
Runner's knee (chondromalacia pa-
    tella), 13, 21, 23, 24, 26–29,
    94, 157, 159–162, 172, 193,
    205, 213, 215, 236–237,
    265, 268
Running, 4, 26, 28, 35–36, 50, 52,
    103, 104, 108, 142–144,
    146, 149, 155–167
    body check, 156–157
    common injuries, 160–164
    conditioning, 158
    gender-related problems, 157
    medical advice, 164–166
    shoes, 159
    tips for, 166–167
    training errors, 160, 162

Salicin, 80
Salter, Robert, 253–254
Sayers, Gale, 3
Second opinions, 68–69, 88
Shinsplints (stress fractures), 24, 50–53,
    159
shoes, 140–146
    aerobic dance, 171
    orthotics, 34, 36, 140, 145–146,
        159, 161, 173, 178, 219
    running, 159
Skating, 4, 238, 241, 242
Skiing, 3, 35, 45, 120, 176–188, 238

bindings, 176, 180–183, 186
    body check, 178–179
    boots, 177, 183–184
    common injuries, 184–185
    conditioning, 179–180, 186
    cross-country, 185–187
    downhill, 176–177, 187
    tips for, 188
Soccer, 4, 238, 241
Soft (low-impact) aerobics, 171,
    173–175
Sounds in knee, 22–23, 59, 233
Spontaneous osteonecrosis, 39–40
Sprains, 44–49, 192–193
Squash, 35
Stabler, Ken, 123
Stair climbing, 9, 31, 105, 107, 153
Stamford, Bryant, 153
Straight-leg raises, 158
Strengthening exercises, 128, 129–130,
    151, 158, 264–269
Stress fractures, 24, 50–53, 159
Stress X rays, 238
Stretching, 14, 15, 148–150, 259–264
Subluxation, 22, 29–32, 193, 234–236
Subotnick, Steven, 178, 179
Sulphasalazine, 133
Supination, 139–140
Surgery:
    arthritis and, 133–135
    information on, 67–69
    meniscus and, 8–9, 42–43, 93,
        253–254
    pros and cons of, 87–89
    rehabilitation and, 101–102
    (see also Arthroscopy; specific
        procedures)
Swelling (effusion), 17–19, 76, 231,
    232, 235
Swimming, 108, 112–113, 129, 130,
    212–214, 241
Synovectomy, 97, 133–134
Synovial fluid, 8
Synovitis, 134, 210
Systemic lupus erythematosus (lupus),
    57–58

Teitz, Carol, 122
Tendinitis, 24, 219
    Achilles', 159
    patellar (jumper's knee), 11, 24,
        33–35, 164, 172–173, 192,
        215
    popliteal, 163–164
Tendon replacement, 252
Tennis (see Racket sports)

Tennis elbow, 217–219
Tenodesis, 119
Terrible triad, 49–50
Tibia, 6, 29
Torn cartilage (*see* Meniscus)
Torn ligaments, 44–49
Total knee arthroplasty (TKA), 9, 40,
    96–99, 134–135
Track and field, 241, 242
Training (*see* Conditioning)
Transcutaneous electrical nerve stimula-
    tion (TENS), 110
Transcutaneous Muscle Stimulation
    (TMS), 110
Traumatic fractures, 50–52
Tulane University, 144

Ulcers, 85
Ultrasound, 109
University of Arizona, 252
University of Cape Town Medical
    School, 162
University of Notre Dame, 216
University of Oregon, 146
University of Virginia, 131
Uric acid, 57, 58

Vastus medialus muscles, 31
Vitamin C, 81
Volleyball, 11, 34

Walking, 130, 141, 144
Warm-up, 149, 150
    (*See also* Exercises)
Water on the knee, 18
Water workouts, 112–113, 129, 130
Weight lifting, 26, 35, 214–217
    body check, 215
    common injuries, 215–216
    overuse injuries, 216–217
    tips for, 217
Weight training, 112, 179–180,
    267–269
Whip kick, 212–214
Whirlpools, 109
Wraps, 34, 118, 123–124
Wrestling, 206–209, 241
    common injuries, 207–208
    conditioning and rehabilitation, 208–209
    tips for, 209

X rays, 51, 58, 74, 75, 235
    stress, 238

Dr. James Fox is a pioneer in the development of sports medicine and the use of arthroscopy, the breakthrough diagnostic and surgical procedure for the knee and other joints. His many past positions include medical director for the Center for the Disorders of the Knee in Van Nuys, California, Orthopedic Consultant for the Denver Gold USFL football team, and member of the medical staff for the 1984 Summer Olympics in Los Angeles. He is currently affiliated with Valley Presbyterian Hospital in Van Nuys, California.

Rick McGuire is a veteran medical writer whose work, for both professional and lay audiences, is translated into eight languages by the International Medical Tribune Syndicate. He is also a frequent contibutor to many consumer publications, including *Health, Total Health, Woman's World,* and the *Los Angeles Times.* After fourteen years in broadcasting, he is currently the Los Angeles correspondent for Physicians Radio Network.